C000229545

BIOCHEMICAL INVESTI
IN LABORATORY MEDICINE

LABORATORY MEDICINE SERIES

Editors: James Hooper MD FRCPath,
Roy Sherwood MSc DPhil,
William Marshall MA, PhD, FRCP, FRCPath

BIOCHEMICAL INVESTIGATIONS
IN LABORATORY MEDICINE

Julian Barth MD, FRCP, MRCPath
Consultant in Chemical Pathology and Metabolic Medicine
Director, SAS Steroid Centre, Leeds Teaching Hospitals NHS Trust

Gary Butler MD, FRCP, FRCPCH
Consultant Paediatric Endocrinologist, Leeds Teaching Hospitals NHS Trust

Peter Hammond MD, FRCP
Consultant Physician and Diabetologist, Harrogate Healthcare NHS Trust

ACB VENTURE PUBLICATIONS

with generous support from Bayer Diagnostics, DPC and Nichols Institute

ACB VENTURE PUBLICATIONS
Chairman - Roy Sherwood

British Library Cataloguing in Publication Data

A catalogue record for the book is available from the British Library

ISBN 0 902429 34 5 ACB Venture Publications

Printed by KSC Printers Ltd, Tunbridge Wells, Kent

Foreword

In the face of the current plethora of information about the biochemical basis of common diseases, it is easy for the clinical investigator to be overwhelmed by the incresasing number of laboratory tests at his or her disposal. This book provides a practical guide to the investigation of biochemical disorders with a focus on the major metabolic disorders. For each disorder, it gives succinct background information and a few key references and/or web addresses. It employs an easy-to-follow problem-based approach using well-designed algorithms that help guide the reader through the maze of possible options and encourages a logical and thoughtful path towards diagnosis.

It is aimed predominantly at clinical biochemists and junior medical staff who may be faced with a patient with a potential metabolic or endocrine disease and who want to be able to make at least a provisional diagnosis before considering referral to a specialised endocrine centre. There are few things more frustating for patient and specialist than having to repeat tiresome tests that have not provided appropriate information. Even more irksome is the excessive use of invasive tests which are not useful. This volume gives clear guidance on the choice and performance of the key tests.

Drs Barth, Butler and Hammond have compiled an excellent guide that should prove an invaluable companion in the investigation of endocrine and metabolic disorders.

Prof Stephen Franks

Preface

Complex clinical problems usually require a spectrum of laboratory investigations initially to aid diagnosis and subsequently to monitor disease and treatment. This book has been designed to help choose the most appropriate tests for different clinical scenarios. These are approached with algorithms which should be used only as a guide for investigation as patients are individuals who do not take kindly to following rigid flow-charts.

Decision points on these algorithms are based on both clinical observations as well as laboratory tests. Some decisions require complex biochemical tests often requiring administration of inhibitory or stimulatory agents. These are described in protocols along with interpretative advice. Some protocols have absolute values for decision making which are based on assay methods employed by the laboratories at Leeds Teaching Hospitals and can only be used as guidance for users of other laboratories.

We are very grateful to all our colleagues for their helpful advice and support and would particularly wish to thank Prof PH Bayliss, Mr AH Balen, Dr PE Belchetz, Dr MJ Henderson, Dr J Hooper and Dr SM Orme for their specific help with some of the more contentious areas of clinical investigation.

Julian Barth
Gary Butler
Peter Hammond
July 2001

Important Notice
Although ACB Venture Publications has made every effort to ensure the accuracy of the information contained in this book, the responsibility for the patient is ultimately that of the medical practitioner ordering or performing/supervising the investigations. All drugs and intravenous fluids must be prescribed by a registered medical practitioner and administered by an individual authorised to do so.

Contents

Part 1 Investigation algorithms

Safety considerations during endocrine/metabolic tests in children

Any dynamic or provocative test has potential for side effects or adverse reactions, although these are uncommon in experienced hands and if appropriate precautions are taken. Precautions, contraindications and adverse reactions are indicated in the protocols for each test and should be reviewed before any test is undertaken. Important adverse reactions in various tests include:

- hypoglycaemia
- dehydration
- minor reactions to provocative agents e.g. nausea, vomiting
- allergic or anaphylactic reaction to provocative agent
- cannula related complications – blood loss, infection
- hypotension.

To minimize potential adverse events the following should be considered.
- Tests on children should only be performed and supervised in specialised paediatric endocrine centres.
- Staff must have detailed knowledge of the particular test protocol and provocative agents.
- Specialised nursing staff familiar with these tests are essential if they are to be performed safely and give accurate results.
- Tests on children must be performed in an environment where full paediatric emergency resuscitation facilities and experience are available. Deaths and serious morbidity have been reported from such testing in inexperienced hands.
- It may be necessary to adjust protocols for particular individuals or circumstances, and the same protocol cannot automatically be safely applied to all patients. Prior to the test, consideration should be given to any particular customisation or precautions required for the individual patient (see guidelines under individual tests). This should be discussed with the consultant concerned.
- Appropriate laboratory back-up is essential, particularly for tests involving fasting, induction of hypoglycaemia or water deprivation. Facilities are required for immediate glucose monitoring in the testing area.
- A medical officer must always be readily available, and in certain tests e.g. insulin hypoglycaemia test, must be immediately available in the ward.
- Experienced personnel are required to site intravenous cannulae.

References
Shah A, Stanhope R, Matthew D. Hazards of pharmacological tests of growth hormone secretion in childhood. Brit Med J 1992; **304**: 173-4.

Siting an IV cannula for serial blood sampling

Most tests require the insertion of one IV cannula through which provocative agents are administered and/or periodic blood samples drawn. *A large vein in the antecubital fossa is the preferred insertion site.* Occasionally separate infusion and sampling cannulas are required. Butterfly needles are useful for single samples, but are not recommended where multiple samples are to be taken.

Requirements
- Local anaesthetic cream (EMLA cream or patch) for children.
- Largest cannula that is practicable; in children this will be size 22 g or 25 g, in adults a size 18 g.
- Water for skin cleansing.
- Vials of IV saline for flushing the cannula.

IV cannula insertion
Local anaesthetic cream is applied for a minimum of one hour (in children).
Site is cleaned with sterile water.
Cannula is inserted and taped in cross-over fashion with 1 cm Micropore tape.
Cannula is flushed with 2 mL normal saline.

Sampling from IV cannula
All samples are drawn using aseptic technique. Gloves should be worn for protection.

When sampling from a cannula, it is imperative that sufficient void volume be removed before the blood sample for analysis is collected, otherwise the sample will be diluted and spurious results obtained. 0.5 to 1 mL should be withdrawn prior to drawing of the blood sample if a standard T-piece is being used – in infants and young children this can be replaced if volume considerations are critical. Cannulae should be flushed with saline, unless patency difficulties are experienced.

Investigation of hypoglycaemia in infancy/childhood

It is most important to ensure that appropriate samples are collected at the time of the hypoglycaemia. Certain tests should be performed as soon as practically possible, including:

- *fluoride oxalate blood:* free fatty acids, 3-hydroxybutyrate, lactate
- *urine:* organic acids.

Other tests should then follow as indicated either by the clinical presentation or the results of the earlier tests.

- The baby's age, gestational age and birthweight are important considerations. Transient hypoglycaemia is common in low birthweight babies in the first two or three days of life. This is largely due to inadequate glycogen stores.

- Maternal diabetes is also an important cause of neonatal hypoglycaemia.

- Plasma concentrations of metabolic intermediates may be difficult to interpret in very low birthweight babies, due to a naturally impaired ketotic response. These babies also often have disproportionately high activities of circulating insulin. The most reliable indication of inappropriate hyperinsulinism is the glucose infusion rate required to maintain normoglycaemia. Usually this does not exceed 10 mg/kg/min.

- Urine sugar analysis must be interpreted with caution. Children with a carbohydrate intolerance will only have an increased urinary excretion of sugars if there has been recent ingestion.

- *Ketonuria is not a reliable guide to the the presence of ketosis:* ketosis can occur when urine strip tests for ketones are negative. This may occur when there is a relative predominance of 3-hydroxybutyrate over acetoacetate as a result of the hepatic redox state and/or intracellular acidosis.

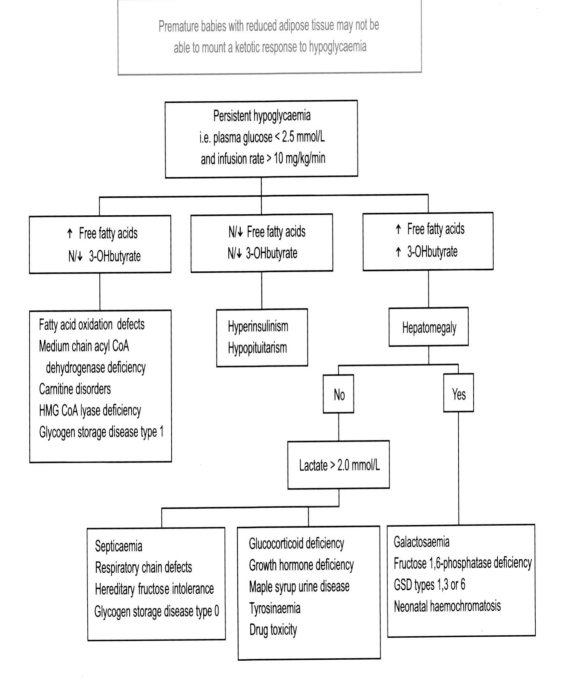

Premature babies with reduced adipose tissue may not be able to mount a ketotic response to hypoglycaemia

Persistent hypoglycaemia
i.e. plasma glucose < 2.5 mmol/L
and infusion rate > 10 mg/kg/min

↑ Free fatty acids
N/↓ 3-OHbutyrate

N/↓ Free fatty acids
N/↓ 3-OHbutyrate

↑ Free fatty acids
↑ 3-OHbutyrate

Fatty acid oxidation defects
Medium chain acyl CoA
    dehydrogenase deficiency
Carnitine disorders
HMG CoA lyase deficiency
Glycogen storage disease type 1

Hyperinsulinism
Hypopituitarism

Hepatomegaly

No

Yes

Lactate > 2.0 mmol/L

Septicaemia
Respiratory chain defects
Hereditary fructose intolerance
Glycogen storage disease type 0

Glucocorticoid deficiency
Growth hormone deficiency
Maple syrup urine disease
Tyrosinaemia
Drug toxicity

Galactosaemia
Fructose 1,6-phosphatase deficiency
GSD types 1,3 or 6
Neonatal haemochromatosis

Investigation of a baby presenting with metabolic acidosis

Before launching into a comprehensive investigation procedure it is necessary to establish that there has been firm evidence of metabolic acidosis i.e. that this was not merely a supposition based on low plasma bicarbonate measurements or hyperventilation. Thereafter, the following clinical information is needed:

- what was the baby's gestational age?
- what is the baby's postnatal age?
- does the baby have respiratory distress?
- was there any evidence of birth asphyxia or traumatic birth?
- how long has the baby been acidotic?
- is the onset or severity of acidosis related to feeding?
- are the baby's parents consanguinous?
- is there a family history of acidosis or neonatal death?

The answers to these questions should influence the way in which an investigation is conducted. A baby presenting with sudden acidosis at several months of age with no prior history is much more likely to have an inborn error of metabolism than a sick, premature baby.

One should bear in mind the old clinical adage that 'common things occur commonly'. That is to say, for most acidotic babies there will be a straightforward aetiology. However, one must be careful not to miss a rare diagnosis being masked by an apparently obvious one. For example, septicaemia is a common complication which can easily cause diagnostic confusion in babies with galactosaemia.

All diagnostic possibilities should be considered until a firm diagnosis has been reached. The presenting features of metabolic diseases are not always consistent between patients. For example, the acute organic acidaemias may not necessarily be associated with marked hyperammonaemia, although this is usually the case. *It is vital that samples are collected at the time that the baby is symptomatic.*

Finally, the complications of acidosis should not be forgotten in the midst of a search for a cause. Hyperkalaemia is a particular danger and unfortunately is often dismissed as factitious when observed in a baby.

The following protocol indicates the important investigations which should lead to a narrower differential diagnosis.

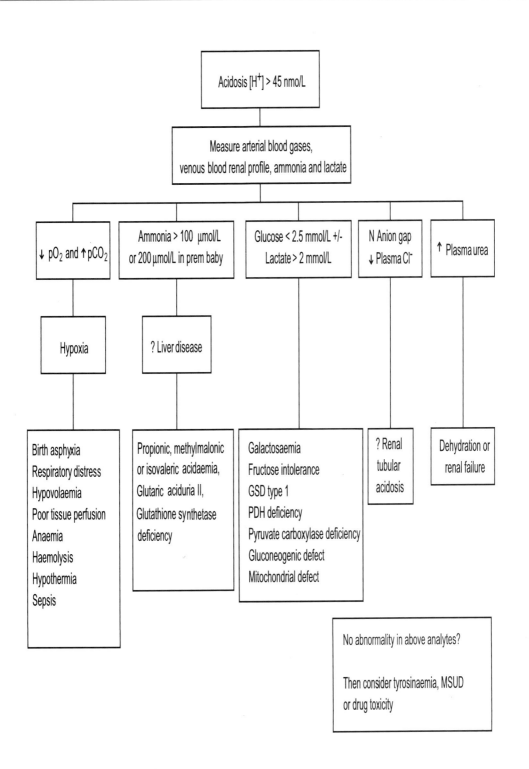

Acidosis [H$^+$] > 45 nmo/L

Measure arterial blood gases,
venous blood renal profile, ammonia and lactate

↓ pO$_2$ and ↑ pCO$_2$

Ammonia > 100 μmol/L
or 200 μmol/L in prem baby

Glucose < 2.5 mmol/L +/-
Lactate > 2 mmol/L

N Anion gap
↓ Plasma Cl$^-$

↑ Plasma urea

Hypoxia

? Liver disease

Birth asphyxia
Respiratory distress
Hypovolaemia
Poor tissue perfusion
Anaemia
Haemolysis
Hypothermia
Sepsis

Propionic, methylmalonic
or isovaleric acidaemia,
Glutaric aciduria II,
Glutathione synthetase
deficiency

Galactosaemia
Fructose intolerance
GSD type 1
PDH deficiency
Pyruvate carboxylase deficiency
Gluconeogenic defect
Mitochondrial defect

? Renal
tubular
acidosis

Dehydration or
renal failure

No abnormality in above analytes?

Then consider tyrosinaemia, MSUD
or drug toxicity

Ambiguous genitalia

A baby born with ambiguous genitalia always causes distress and concern. It has to be emphasised that handling of this situation must be the responsibility of experienced senior staff as major mistakes can occur in the diagnosis and interpretation of results and in the correct assignment of sex. The presence of one or two palpable gonads may help with the interpretation of subsequent results. Chromosomal karyotype is valuable but the genotype is not necessarily a good guide to the decision about the sex of rearing. Because of major changes in the adrenal gland in the first three days of life, it is not helpful to collect a plasma or urine sample until after 72 hours from birth. Gestational age needs to be taken into consideration when interpreting 17-hydroxyprogesterone concentrations as they are much higher in preterm infants. Under-virilisation of a male is of greater consequence than virilisation of a female infant as it is usually more difficult to achieve satisfactory outcome.

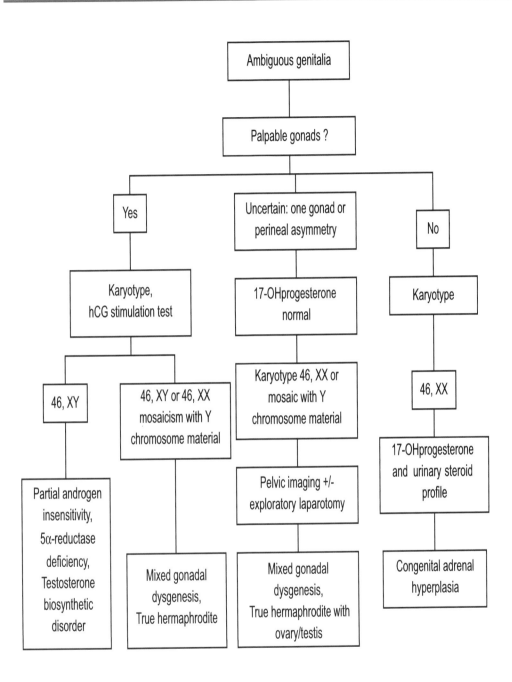

Short stature or delayed growth

The first step in the investigation of a child with short stature is to confirm that the child really is short, since there are frequently serious errors of measurement due to poor technique or poor equipment as well as incorrect entries on growth charts. Another key point is to determine whether the child is shorter than expected in relation to his/her family as a number of conditions can be ruled out when the genetic target height is low.

When a child is noted to be inappropriately short, assessment of body proportion can rule out the small percentage of children with abnormalities of their skeletal architecture following which one can continue with a staged investigation plan. It should be born in mind that endocrine causes of poor growth are relatively rare. In the first instance, systemic or multi-system disease and non-organic conditions such as psychosocial deprivation should be considered. Subsequently, prior to considering full endocrine investigations, it is appropriate to document an abnormally slow growth rate as pituitary function tests are rarely indicated in the presence of normal growth and indeed their interpretation in children with normal growth is very difficult. Normal growth may be defined as more than 5 cm per year in mid-childhood and a significantly abnormal height velocity would be less than 4 cm per year.

The planning and the interpretation of tests of pituitary function and growth hormone secretion requires some forethought. As there is a physiological diminution of growth hormone secretion in the latter part of pre-puberty, the stimulated peak of growth hormone may fall below the recommended cut off (which should be determined locally, based on the specific growth hormone assay). In children with a bone age over 10 years, it is appropriate to pre-treat (prime) with sex steroid therapy. In a boy this can be done with intramuscular Sustanon (testosterone) 100 mg five days before the investigation; in a girl, with oral ethinyloestradiol 10 µg daily for five days prior to the investigation. This upregulates the pituitary gland into increasing growth hormone output into pubertal activity.

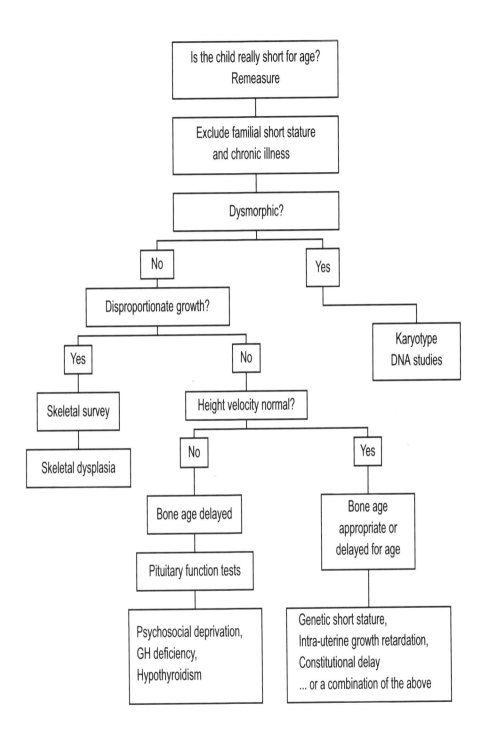

Tall stature

The key issues in determining whether a child with tall stature has a serious medical problem are determining in the first place whether the child is actually considerably taller in relation to his/her parents and secondly whether the child is growing at a normal or accelerated growth rate. Children who are unusually tall for their family and who have body disproportions i.e. long legs or arms, or a big head may have a genetic cause for their tallness. Precocious sexual maturity is usually the cause of rapid growth in a phenotypically normal child as growth hormone excess (gigantism) is extremely rare. Refer to appropriate sections.

In children with normal growth velocity, an advanced bone age gives some prognosis to final height. If bone age is normal for chronological age, the child is likely to have a tall adult height. An advanced bone age suggests that an adult height in keeping with the biological parents will be achieved at an earlier age than normally expected.

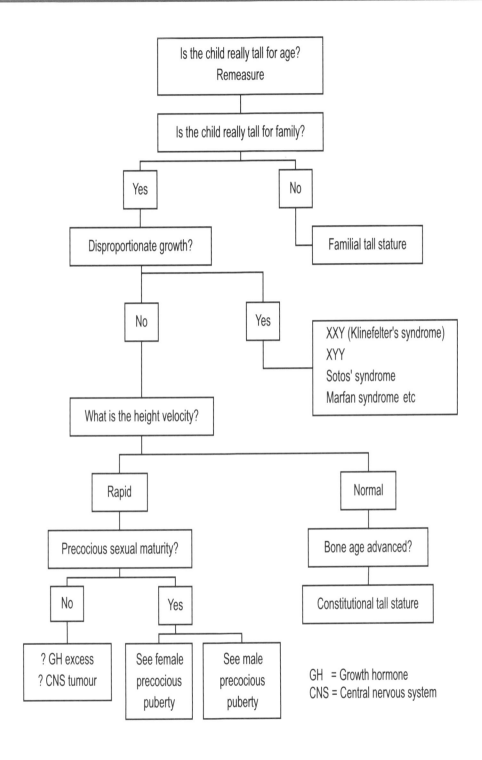

Delayed puberty in females

The commonest cause for delayed sexual development in girls is simple maturational delay but overt or cryptic chronic illnesses may delay the onset of puberty. This is less of a major problem in girls than in boys as the first sign of puberty, namely breast development, is immediately noticeable and is quickly followed by mood changes and very rapid growth. In the absence of breast development, a useful next investigation is pelvic ultrasound which will show follicular changes and ovarian growth if puberty is imminent. If the ovaries are small and pre-pubertal in configuration then raised gonadotrophins will detect primary ovarian failure. Low gonadotrophins may be present in isolated gonadotrophin deficiency or combined genetic syndromes such as Kallman's syndrome but also as a result of intracranial lesions. Eating disorders may significantly delay the onset of puberty and extreme maturational delay can occur.

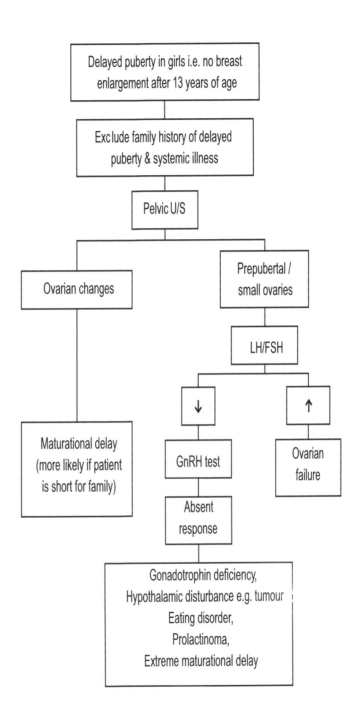

Delayed puberty in males

Unless a patient is examined carefully, the earliest signs of puberty i.e. testicular vascularisation and slight enlargement, may well be missed. The commonest cause of delayed puberty is simple maturational delay but this is a diagnosis of exclusion and other common causes such as systemic or chronic illnesses need to be ruled out. In a normal healthy boy with no signs of puberty, a useful screening test is an 08:00h plasma testosterone concentration. A concentration above 1 nmol/L will indicate the presence of nocturnal pulsatile LH secretion, the first endocrine event initiating puberty. At lower concentrations of testosterone, gonadotrophins are the next appropriate investigation to perform as they are raised in primary testicular failure. The most difficult diagnostic problem is when both testosterone and gonadotrophin concentrations are low; this may be due to an idiopathic isolated deficiency, an intracranial lesion, an associated genetic defect (Kallman's syndrome) or sometimes just extreme maturational delay.

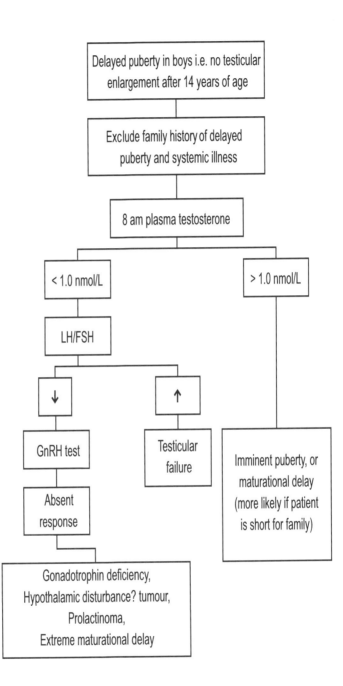

Precocious sexual development in girls

Precocious sexual development is defined as the appearance of secondary sexual maturation before the age of eight years. The direction of investigation can be helped by noting whether or not breast development is present. Breast development signifies oestrogen secretion which is either due to ovarian autonomy (ovarian cyst) or McCune Albright's syndrome (gonadotrophin-independent puberty), or initiation of the normal pubertal mechanism (gonadotrophin-dependent puberty). In girls precocious sexual development is most often idiopathic but can arise from CNS disturbance such as intracranial lesions, hydrocephaly and head injuries.

Signs of sexual development (pubic and axillary hair, rapid growth, acne and body odour) without breast enlargement are usually due to adrenal androgens. The commonest cause is simple precocious adrenarche, a normal variant occurring between six and seven years of age, but adrenal pathology (tumours, late onset congenital adrenal hyperplasia, etc.) must be excluded.

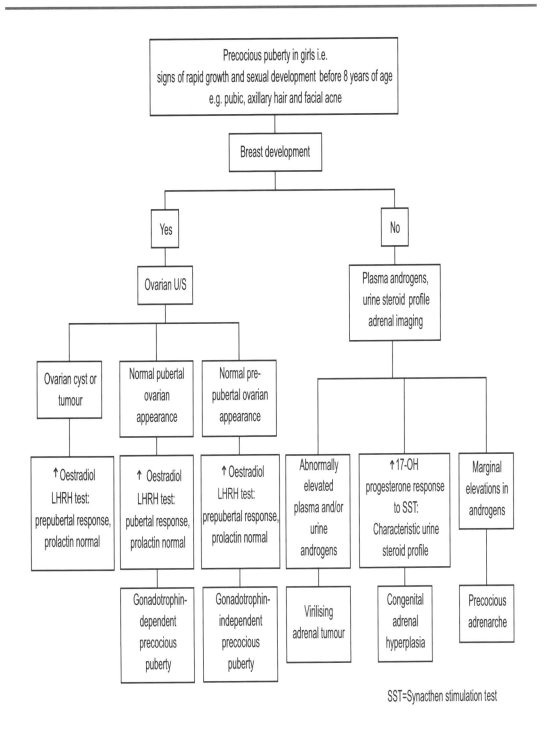

Precocious sexual development in boys

In boys who present with signs of sexual development before the age of nine, the key to further investigation and the diagnosis is the demonstration of testicular enlargement. If this is present, there is usually abnormal pubertal gonadotrophin secretion often secondary to a CNS tumour (gonadotrophin-dependent precocious puberty). Primary hypothyroidism can, however, rarely present in this way. In the absence of testicular enlargement, one needs to exclude pathological causes from normal variations. Adrenarche, which occurs in boys on average at seven years, is a normal variant and may cause some pubic hair growth. The source of excess androgens is usually adrenal as auto-regulation of the testes (testotoxicosis) is extremely rare (gonadotrophin-independent precocious puberty).

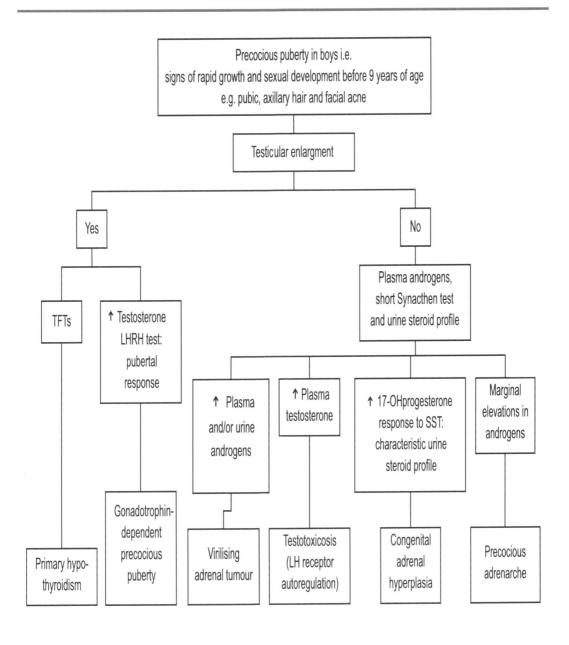

SST= Synacthen stimulation test

TFT= Thyroid function tests

Cushing's syndrome

Cushing's syndrome may be ACTH-dependent, due to a pituitary tumour or an ectopic source, or ACTH-independent due to an adrenal tumour.

There are two different patterns of ACTH-dependent Cushing's syndrome. Cushing's disease is due to a pituitary adenoma secreting ACTH. It is an indolent condition, which may present with any of a plethora of features: typical facies, obesity, proximal myopathy, secondary diabetes, hypertension, hypogonadism, osteoporosis, purple striae, hirsuties and acne, ankle oedema and buffalo hump. Following the diagnosis, the disease can often be retrospectively detected from old photographs which may show that clinical signs have been present for many years.

Ectopic ACTH can be secreted by a tiny (and often unlocalisable) benign tumour which mimics the natural history of a pituitary adenoma. However, secretion from malignant tumours results in a metabolic condition of excessive mineralocorticoid action with predominant muscle weakness due to hypokalaemic alkalosis with plasma potassium often < 2.0 mmol/L. These patients are usually thin and deeply pigmented and have an extremely poor prognosis with a 50% survival of only a few weeks.

Diagnostic strategy

Cushing's syndrome is one of the most difficult problems in clinical endocrinology. It is frequently suspected but rarely diagnosed. There are two phases to investigation: first, the diagnosis of hypercortisolism and second, the localisation of the source. For the former, we propose an overnight dexamethasone suppression test and 24 hour urinary cortisol as screening tests. This combination has a relatively high false positive rate but false negatives are very rare. The localisation of the source of ACTH may be extremely difficult and it is probably appropriate to refer patients to an endocrinologist when non-suppressible cortisol has been demonstrated; for this reason we have not included a protocol for the low dose dexamethasone suppression test. Following the confirmation of hypercortisolism, adrenal causes are best detected by imaging techniques.

If the diagnosis is strongly suspected and the screening tests are negative, the diagnosis should not be discounted as there are well recorded cases of cyclical Cushing's disease with episodes of clinical and biochemical normality between episodes of typical clinical and biochemical disease.

Diagnostic tests for Cushing's syndrome

	Sensitivity	Specificity
Urinary free cortisol (UFC)	95-100 %	98 %
1 mg dexamethasone suppression test	98-100 %	80 %

	False positives	False negatives
UFC	Physical stress e.g. trauma, exercise, malnutrition Mental stress e.g. depression, alcohol or drug abuse/withdrawal Metabolic e.g. raised cortisol binding globulin (CBG), glucocorticoid resistance, complicated diabetes	Renal failure Inadequate collection
1mg dexamethasone suppression test	Depression Severe systemic illness Renal failure on dialysis Chronic alcohol abuse Old age Anorexia nervosa Hepatic enzyme inducing drugs e.g. rifampicin, phenytoin Drugs which increase CBG e.g. HRT, oral contraceptives, tamoxifen	Very rare in patients with Cushing's disease – if clinical suspicion is high continue investigating

Reference
Wood P, Barth JH, Freedman DB, Perry L, Sheridan B. Evidence for the low dose dexamethasone suppression test to screen for Cushing's syndrome – recommendations for a protocol for UK biochemistry laboratories. Ann Clin Biochem 1997; **34:** 222-9.

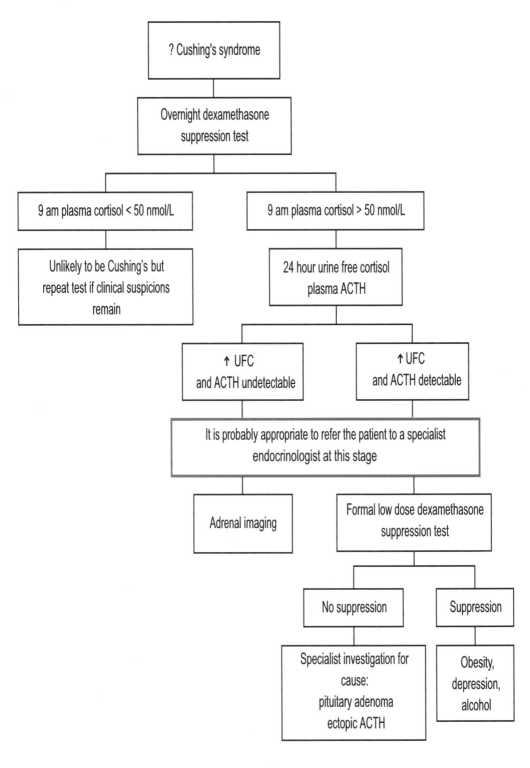

Hyperprolactinaemia

Hyperprolactinaemia is physiological during pregnancy and lactation. With these exceptions, the commonest non-drug causes of hyperprolactinaemia are stress, microprolactinomas, polycystic ovary syndrome and primary hypothyroidism. Women present with infertility, galactorrhoea or menstrual irregularities and, rarely, with the mass effect of tumour extending outside the pituitary fossa. In men, tumours tend to be larger at presentation, which is either with sexual dysfunction or features related to the space-occupying effect of the tumours.

The normal pattern of prolactin in pregnancy is for a gradual rise in plasma concentration during the first two trimesters followed by a brisk rise in the third trimester to 6000-10,000 mU/L. Prolactin remains elevated during lactation but gradually falls to normal with prolonged breast feeding.

Notes

• Prolactin may be elevated in patients with renal or liver disease but this should not alter management regarding the need to image the pituitary gland.

• The choice of 800 mU/L as a threshold for imaging the pituitary is a compromise and will be affected by clinical features; for example, in women with galactorrhoea/oligomenorrhoea use a sustained value greater than 600 mU/L whereas in asymptomatic patients a threshold of 1000 mU/L may be more appropriate.

• Stress is a recognised cause of mild hyperprolactinaemia and under these circumstances repeated samples, taken through an indwelling cannula over an hour will show a fall.

• Prior to investigating patients for pituitary tumours, hypothyroidism should always be excluded as a cause of hyperprolactinaemia.

• Hyperprolactinaemia may be the result of macro forms of prolactin due to complexes with immunoglobulins and not to a pituitary tumour.

Drugs causing hyperprolactinaemia

Dopamine receptor agonists

Neuroleptics

Anti-emetics: metoclopramide, domperidone

Selective serotonin reuptake inhibitors (SSRIs)

Tricyclic antidepressants (rare)

Cardiovascular drugs: verapamil, reserpine, methyldopa

High dose oestrogens

Opiates

Miscellaneous: bezafibrate, omeprazole, trimethoprim, histamine H2 antagonists

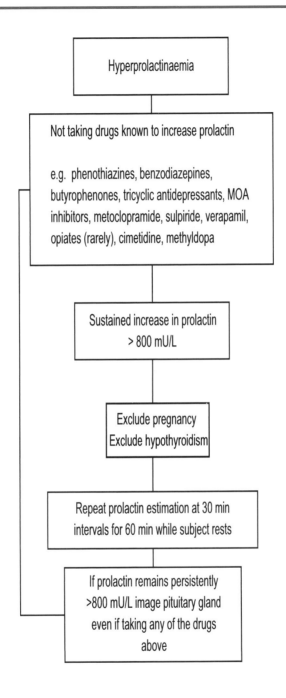

Biochemical investigation of a pituitary incidentaloma

The advent of high quality pituitary imaging has led to the recognition of unsuspected pituitary tumours. This is not surprising since autopsy studies have shown that 10-20% normal individuals have pituitary microadenomas. The most frequently occuring tumours (> 80%) are prolactinomas and non-functioning tumours. Other tumours, aneurysms and inflammation may also present as a tumour on imaging.

The following tests should be carried out:

• Random measurement of gonadotrophins, TFTs, prolactin and glycoprotein alpha subunits.

• Screening tests for cortisol hypersecretion by 24 h urine free cortisol and 1mg overnight dexamethasone suppression test.

• Screening for excess growth hormone (page 148).

Reference
Molitch ME. Evaluation and treatment of the patient with a pituitary incidentaloma. J Clin Endocrinol Metab 1995; **80**: 3-6.

Hypopituitarism

Pituitary reserve is completely assessed by using a combined pituitary function test: this combines an insulin hypoglycaemia test (IHT), TRH and GnRH tests. In practice the TRH and GnRH tests provide no clinically useful information above that provided by basal hormone measurements of TFTs, gonadotrophins, prolactin and gonadal steroids. Moreover, there are case reports of pituitary apoplexy associated with the use of both TRH and GnRH.

The IHT causes stress-related release of cortisol and GH by the effects of insulin induced hypoglycaemia. It is contraindicated in individuals over age 70, and those with ischaemic heart disease or epilepsy, and is unpleasant in all cases.

Alternatives to the IHT are the glucagon stimulation test, which induces release of both GH and cortisol, and is thus comparable to the ITT, or the short Synacthen test, which has the disadvantage of only testing adrenal reserve not the whole pituitary-adrenal axis.

Reference
Burke CW. The pituitary megatest: outdated? Clin Endocrinol (Oxf) 1992; **36**: 133-4.

Suspected adrenal failure

Patients with adrenal failure may present acutely, with hypoglycaemia or hyponatraemia and hypovolaemia, or chronically with general malaise, anorexia, vomiting, intermittent abdominal pain and weight loss. Signs of hypovolaemia include hypotension, often postural, and tachycardia. Pigmentation is seen on sun-exposed areas and also sites of friction such as the palmar creases, elbows, knuckles and buccal mucosa.

If the diagnosis is strongly suspected, there should be no delay in administering glucocorticoids as soon as blood has been taken for plasma cortisol and ACTH; the definitive diagnosis can wait. If dexamethasone is given, the short Synacthen test can be performed the next day as dexamethasone does not interfere with cortisol assays.

Care should be taken in interpreting the short Synacthen test in women taking an oral contraceptive since elevations in cortisol binding globulin will result in high basal and stimulated cortisol concentrations.

Patients given long term corticosteroid therapy will have become hypoadrenal due to adrenal atrophy. As a result they may have a poor response to exogenous ACTH, but there is no evidence that the response to ACTH is useful in tailoring glucocorticoid withdrawal. If they appear to have inappropriate symptoms and concern persists about their adrenal reserve, it is probably better to evaluate the entire hypothalamo-adrenal axis e.g. by using an i.m. glucagon test.

References
Clarke PMS, Neylon I, Raggatt PR, Sheppard MC, Stewart PM. Defining the normal cortisol response to the short Synacthen test: implications for the investigation of hypothalamo-pituitary disorders. Clin Endocrinol (Oxf) 1998; **49**: 287-92.

Ostlere LS, Rumsby G, Holownia P, Jacobs HS, Rustin HA, Honour JW. Carrier status for steroid 21-hydroxylase deficiency is only one factor in the variable phenotype of acne. Clin Endocrinol (Oxf) 1998; **48**: 209-15.

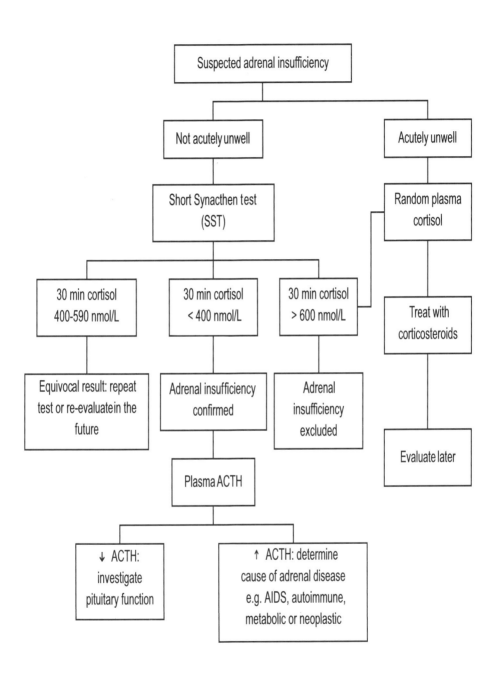

Suspected phaeochromocytoma

Catecholamine-secreting tumours are rare and as many as 50% are diagnosed at post mortem. The clinical features described are of episodic or uncontrollable and sustained hypertension and/or symptoms of sympathetic overactivity e.g. sweating, palpitation, pallor and headache. However, many patients with phaeochromocytoma diagnosed during work-up or follow-up of multiple endocrine neoplasia (MEN) syndromes are asymptomatic.

The diagnosis is based on increased urinary catecholamine excretion. Two consecutive 24 hour urine collections are recommended in order to ensure that patients with episodic secretion are detected. Urine collections must be made into containers containing acid to ensure preservation of catecholamines. Plasma catecholamine measurement is not recommended in routine practice in view of the false positive stress response, but may be helpful in patients with poor urine output or for localisation of extra-adrenal tumours.

The optimal diagnostic protocol is to measure both free catecholamines and their metabolites, the metanephrines. Some antihypertensive agents may interfere with the analytical methods and the laboratory should be contacted for advice.

Reference
Lips CJ, Landsvater RM, Hoppener JW, Geerdink RA, Blijham G, van Veen JM, van Gils AP, de Wit MJ, Zewald RA, Berends MJ. Clinical screening as compared with DNA analysis in families with multiple endocrine neoplasia type 2A. New Engl J Med 1994; **331:** 828-35.

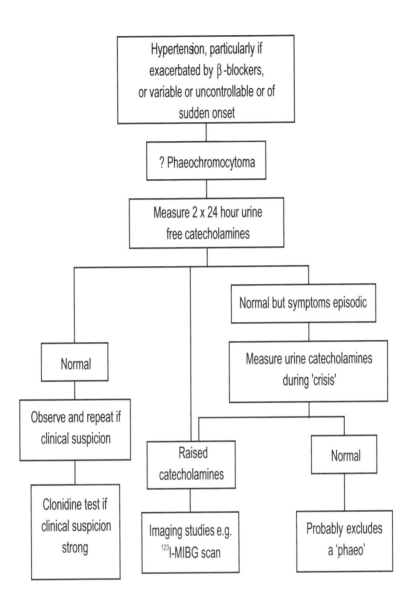

Hyperaldosteronism

Does the patient have hyperaldosteronism?

Spontaneous or diuretic-induced hypokalaemia has traditionally been considered a useful diagnostic guide to hyperaldosteronism in hypertensive patients. However, it has become apparent that up to 50% of subjects with primary hyperaldosteronism are normokalaemic. Moreover, ACE inhibitors used for the treatment of hypertension may elevate plasma potassium and might disguise underlying hyperaldosteronism. Therefore a high degree of clinical suspicion is required for diagnosis and hypokalaemia can no longer be considered a sufficiently sensitive diagnostic tool.

The use of random aldosterone/renin ratios as a first line test is becoming more established and is probably less affected by drug therapy, diurnal variation and patient position than either aldosterone or renin alone. The use of a ratio also helps to diagnose those subjects with early adenomatous hyperaldosteronism in whom the renin is suppressed but with only a marginally elevated plasma aldosterone concentration.

Once the diagnosis of primary hyperaldosteronism has been made, it is then necessary to establish the cause. The commonest cause is an adrenal tumour (adenoma or carcinoma) and pre-operative localisation is necessary as tumours visualised on imaging are not always functional. Other causes include idiopathic hyperaldosteronism and glucocorticoid-suppressible hyperaldosteronism. Conditions mimicking the clinical presentation of hyperaldosteronism include: SAME (syndromes of apparent mineralocorticoid excess), liquorice abuse, Cushing's syndrome, congenital adrenal hyperplasia (11β- or 17α-hydroxylase deficiency), Liddle's syndrome (mutation of β subunit of epithelial sodium channel), syndromes of cortisol resistance and deoxycorticosterone producing adrenal tumours.

References

Gordon RD. Mineralocorticoid hypertension. Lancet 1994; **344:** 240-3.

McKenna TJ, Sequiera SJ, Heffernan A, Chambers J, Cunningham S. Diagnosis under random conditions of all disorders of the renin-aldosterone axis, including primary hyperaldosteronism. J Clin Endocrinol Metab 1991; **73:** 952-7.

Valloton MB. Primary hyperaldosteronism. Part I Diagnosis of primary hyperaldosteronism. Clin Endocrinol 1996; **45:** 47-52.

Valloton MB. Primary hyperaldosteronism. Part II Differential diagnosis of primary hyperaldosteronism and pseudoaldosteronism. Clin Endocrinol 1996; **45:** 53-60.

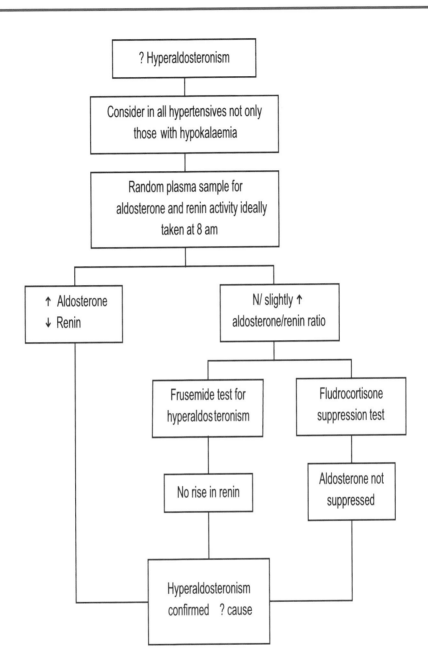

? Hyperaldosteronism

Consider in all hypertensives not only those with hypokalaemia

Random plasma sample for aldosterone and renin activity ideally taken at 8 am

↑ Aldosterone
↓ Renin

N/ slightly ↑ aldosterone/renin ratio

Frusemide test for hyperaldosteronism

Fludrocortisone suppression test

No rise in renin

Aldosterone not suppressed

Hyperaldosteronism confirmed   ? cause

Biochemical investigation of an adrenal incidentaloma

The advent of high quality abdominal imaging has led to the recognition of unsuspected adrenal tumours. The majority of these tumours are silent or only express subtle forms of hypercortisolism. However, since the morbidity associated with adrenal nodules is related to hormonal hypersecretion or malignancy, patients in whom such tumours have been identified should be investigated for hitherto unsuspected and overt hormonal hypersecretion, sub-clinical hormonal hypersecretion or primary or secondary adrenal malignancy (imaging and/or fine needle biopsy).

The following tests should be carried out:

• screening tests for cortisol hypersecretion by 24 h urinary free cortisol and 1mg overnight dexamethasone suppression test

• screening for phaeochromocytoma (page 32)

• screening for hyperaldosteronism (page 34)

• screening for excess androgen secretion (page 44).

References

Osella G, Terzolo M, Borretta G, Magro G, Ali A, Piovesan A, Paccotti P, Angeli A. Endocrine evaluation of incidentally discovered adrenal masses (incidentalomas). J Clin Endocrinol Metab 1994; **79:** 1532-9.

Tsagarakis A. The management of adrenal incidentalomas. In: Grossman A (ed). Clinical Endocrinology 2nd edit. Blackwells Science, Oxford 1998: 484-93.

Abnormal thyroid function tests

Thyroid dysfunction may cause relatively non-specific symptoms such as fatigue, malaise, mood swings, bowel disturbance and palpitation. Whilst the classically thyrotoxic or hypothyroid patient can be diagnosed clinically, thyroid function tests are commonly performed in patients experiencing non-specific symptoms without convincing signs of thyroid disease, and similarly the biochemical picture is not always typical.

The predictive value of abnormalities in thyroid function are derived from a community based study in North England – the 'Whickham Survey'. This demonstrated that the annual incidence of hypothyroidism was 3.5/1000 women. The odds ratio for developing hypothyroidism were:

8 for women and 44 for men with an isolated increase in TSH
8 for women and 25 for men with positive anti-thyroid antibodies
38 for women and 173 for men with an increase in TSH and positive antibodies.

Positive thyroid microsomal antibodies were present in 21% of women aged 55-65 years and these women had an annual risk of developing hypothyroidism of 2.6%.

Over 20 years one third of women with an isolated increase in TSH will become clinically hypothyroid.

Hyperthyroidism is much less common with an annual incidence of 0.8/1000 women. It is even less common in men.

Isolated suppressed TSH may occasionally indicate early hyperthyroidism. However, treatment is probably only of benefit in such patients if there is associated atrial fibrillation.

Interpretation of thyroid function tests in the elderly can be problematical. TSH may be suppressed in normal elderly subjects and thyroid biochemistry is particularly susceptible to intercurrent illness in elderly people, although a 'sick euthyroid' pattern can be seen in any patient with significant acute illness. The commonest abnormality is a decrease in thyroid hormone concentrations with normal TSH; the fall is more marked with total than 'free' hormones and for T3 than T4. During recovery there is a delayed rise in TSH, which may rise above the reference range, as thyroid hormone concentrations return to normal. However, any change in TSH concentration may be seen in association with non-thyroidal illness. The best advice is not to test thyroid function in an acutely unwell patient unless there is a strong clinical suspicion of thyroid dysfunction, especially since giving thyroid hormone to patients with non-thyroidal illness has not been shown to be of benefit.

Drugs affecting TSH concentration

Decrease TSH	Increase TSH
bromocriptine	clomiphene
carbamazepine	iodides
corticosteroids	lithium
cyproheptadine	metoclopramide
dopamine	morphine
heparin	phenothiazines
levodopa	
thyroxine, tri-iodothyronine	

References

Vanderpump MP, Tunbridge WM, French JM, Appleton D, Bates D, Clark F, Grimley Evans J, Hasan DM, Rodgers H, Tunbridge F, et al. The incidence of thyroid disorders in the community: a twenty-year follow-up of the Whickham Survey. Clin Endocrinol (Oxf) 1995; **43:** 55-68.

Rae P, Farrar J, Beckett G, Toft A. Assessment of thyroid status in elderly people Brit Med J 1993; **307:** 177-80.

Sawin CT, Geller A, Wolf PA, Belanger AJ, Baker E, Bacharach P, Wilson PWF, Benjamin EJ, D'Agostino RB. Low serum thyrotropin concentrations as a risk factor or atrial fibrillation in older persons. New Engl J Med 1994; **331:** 1249-52.

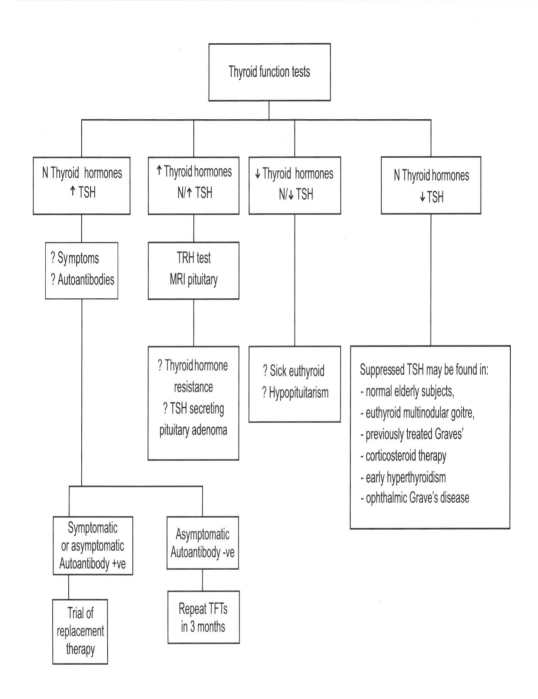

Excessive body hair growth

Hirsutism

Hirsutism is defined as hair growth in a woman on the face and body which appears in the same pattern and with the same temporal development as in men. This form of hair growth is dependent on stimulation by androgens. It differs significantly from *hypertrichosis* which is an uniform growth of hair over the entire body and which develops either as part of a congenital or metabolic disorder (e.g. anorexia nervosa and hypothyroidism) or in response to non-hormonal drugs (e.g. cyclosporin and minoxidil).

The presence of hirsutism can only be determined by clinical examination of the pattern and timing of the hair growth. The natural development of androgenic body hair begins at puberty with a conversion of vellus to terminal hairs in the pubic area followed by the axillae after an interval of about two years. Facial hair appears at the same time as axillary hair in boys. Terminal hairs start at the corners of the lips and spread over the upper lip before appearing on the chin and then cheeks. An orderly sequence of hair conversion follows on the body: the lower legs, thighs, forearms, abdomen, buttocks, chest, back, upper arms and shoulders.

Hypertrichosis

Hypertrichosis differs first in having an uniform distribution of hair over the entire body and second as the hair shafts themselves have an homogeneous silky smooth form unlike the thick, coarse and curly hair shafts seen in hirsutism.

Investigation strategy for hirsuties

A full clinical evaluation should be made for the pattern of development of hirsuties and the presence of systemic virilism (i.e. cliteromegaly, increased muscle bulk, deep voice, scalp balding, amenorrhoea, etc.). In the absence of features of systemic virilism, a measurement of plasma testosterone is a suitable screening test for serious endocrine disturbance. Further evaluation is required if the testosterone is >5 nmol/L in premenopausal or >3 nmol/L in post-menopausal women. Investigations to evaluate the degree of insulin resistance such as fasting glucose and lipid profile may also be appropriate.

References

Barth JH. Investigations in the assessment and management of patients with hirsutism. Curr Opin Obstet Gynaecol 1997; **10:** 187-92.

Reynolds EL. The appearance of adult patterns of body hair in man. Ann NY Acad Sci 1951; **53:** 576-84.

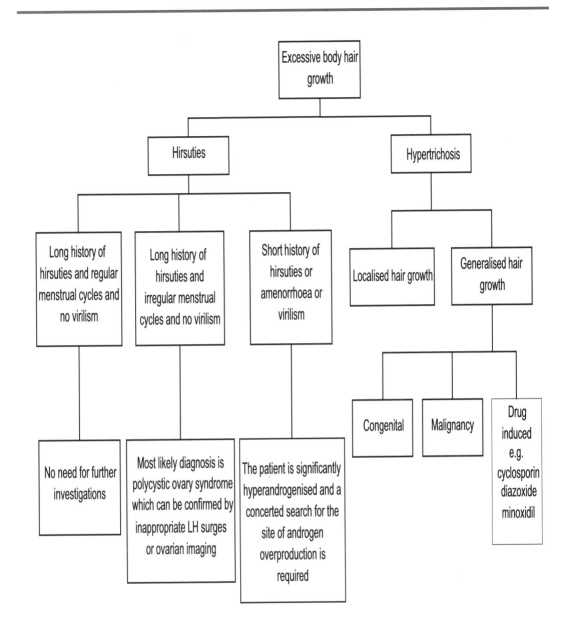

A/oligomenorrhoea and infertility

When couples present with infertility both partners require evaluation. If semen analysis is abnormal, an endocrine profile, including testosterone and gonadotrophins will be required from the male partner. Women with regular periods are unlikely to have an endocrine problem. A luteal phase progesterone measurement is probably *not* necessary (see below). Rarely, hyperprolactinaemia may cause anovulation in women with regular cycles, but far more often there is associated menstrual disturbance.

Polycystic ovary syndrome is a clinical diagnosis, women presenting with any of acne, hirsutism, oligomenorrhoea and subfertility. Transvaginal ultrasound, particularly when performed by an experienced operator, may corroborate the clinical impression.

Midluteal progesterone

Since women with regular cycles (30+/- 2 days) ovulate in 95% of those cycles, progesterone measurement is probably unnecessary. Blood samples for progesterone need to be taken at the mid luteal point, which is 7 days prior to the onset of the next menstrual bleed. Therefore, in women who are cycling regularly, the commonest cause of a low progesterone (< 30 nmol/L) is likely to be due to inaccurate sample timing. High concentrations of progesterone i.e. > 100 nmol/L may indicate early pregnancy.

FSH for prediction of fertility

Measurement of plasma FSH on day 3 can give some guide to the odds for successful conception. If the FSH > 8 IU/L there is a reduced likelihood of conception; this becomes very small when FSH > 15 IU/L.

Monitoring women with erratic cycles

In women with erratic cycles, it may be more appropriate to co-ordinate endocrine tests with ultrasound monitoring of ovarian activity.

References

Hull MGR, Savage PE, Bromham DR, Ismail AAA, Morris FA. The value of a single serum progesterone measurement in the midluteal phase as a criterion of a potentially fertile cycle ("ovulation") derived from treated and untreated conception cycles. Fertil Steril 1982; **37**: 355-60.

Kyei-Mensah AA, Jacobs HS. The investigation of female infertility. Clin Endocrinol (Oxf) 1995; **43**: 251-5.

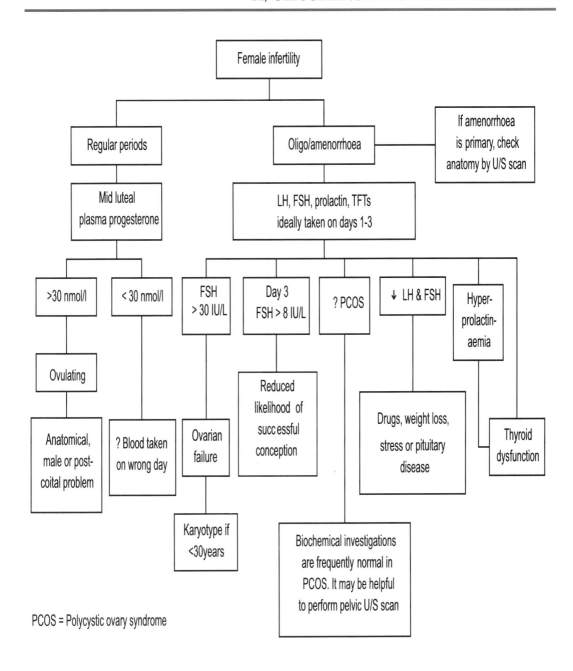

PCOS = Polycystic ovary syndrome

Investigation of female virilism

The most difficult decision in the management of women with hyperandrogenism e.g. acne, hirsuties, polycystic ovaries, etc. is when exhaustive investigation should be instituted. Since the treatment of hirsute women presenting with non-tumourous hyperandrogenism will be similar whether the androgen is from the adrenals or ovaries, it is only necessary to identify those women with an androgen secreting tumour. This chart suggests the criteria for investigation should be the presence of any of the following features: an elevated random plasma testosterone concentration, a short history of hirsuties or features of systemic virilism e.g. cliteromegaly, increased muscle bulk, deep voice, androgenic alopecia or amenorrhoea.

Evidence for identification of androgen secreting tumours

Derksen *et al* reported a series of two adrenal adenomas and 12 carcinomas in which hirsutism was the presenting symptom. The women with adenomas were described as being severely virilised. Half of the women with carcinoma had clinical signs of Cushing's syndrome; of the remaining six, four were severely virilised and the other two women presented with abdominal pain.

Functioning ovarian tumours that secrete androgens and therefore cause virilisation are rare and represent only 1% of all ovarian tumours. In these cases, hirsuties is a nearly universal feature. Amenorrhoea develops rapidly in all premenopausal patients and systemic virilisation with alopecia, cliteromegaly, deepening of the voice and a male habitus develops in about half of the patients. Meldrum and Abraham reviewed 43 women with virilising ovarian tumours: seven had plasma testosterone < 7.0 nmol/L but all were clinically virilised; one 65 year-old woman was reported as not virilised but her plasma testosterone was > 12 nmol/L.

Patients with androgen secreting tumours can therefore be detected by a combination of a good history and examination and a plasma testosterone measurement.

References

Derksen J, Nagesser Sk, Meinders AE, Haak HR, van de Velde CJH. Identification of virilising adrenal tumours in hirsute women. N Eng J Med 1994; **331**: 968-73.

Friedman CI, Schmidt GE, Kim MH, Powell J. Serum testosterone concentrations in the evaluation of androgen-producing tumors. Am J Obstet Gynecol 1985; **153**: 44-9.

Meldrum DR, Abraham GE. Peripheral and ovarian venous concentration of various steroid hormones in virilising ovarian tumours. Obstet Gynecol 1979; **53**: 36-43.

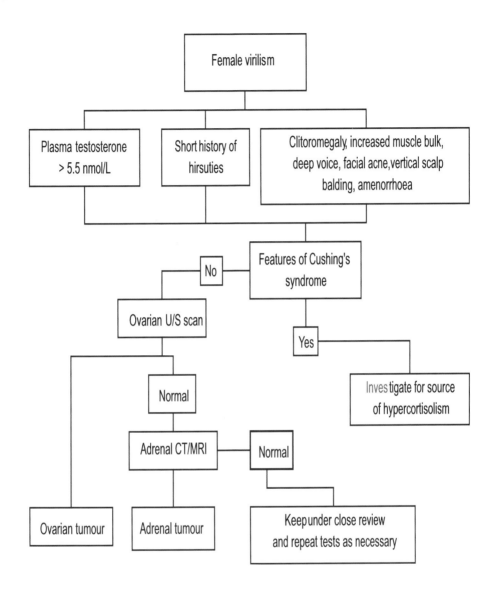

Gynaecomastia

Gynaecomastia is the enlargement of glandular tissue of the breast and should be distinguished from an increase in adipose tissue. It is usually bilateral, but may be strikingly asymmetrical, or unilateral. It results from an increase in the effective oestrogen: androgen ratio within the mammary tissue.

Physiological gynaecomastia can occur at the extremes of life, but is most common during puberty, when it usually lasts for only a few months, although may persist into adulthood.

The index of suspicion and therefore the need for endocrine investigation of gynaecomastia will depend on the age of the subject and findings on detailed history and physical examination. Pathological gynaecomastia is likely when sudden enlargement occurs unrelated to puberty, particularly in young boys or middle aged men. The most common identifiable cause is drug therapy, but there is no obvious aetiology in up to 50% of cases.

Initial steps should include a detailed drug history. A positive drug history cannot exclude a breast cancer which should always be considered, especially in the elderly. Endocrine investigations should be considered if gynaecomastia is persistent or progressive.

The underlying cause in the majority of cases will be an imbalance in the functional ratio between androgens and oestrogens. Altered breast tissue response may be considered if all other identifiable causes are excluded.

Reference
Ismail AAA, Barth JH. The endocrinology of gynaecomastia. Ann Clin Biochem 2001 In Press

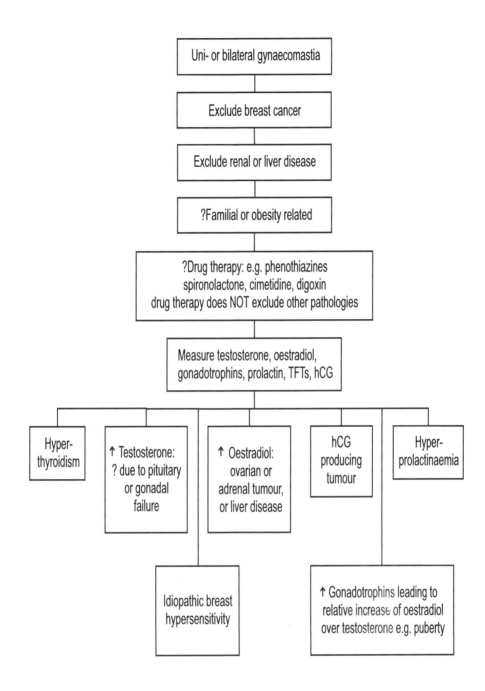

Diabetes mellitus

WHO Diagnostic criteria 2001

1. Symptoms of diabetes (i.e. polyuria, polydipsia and unexplained weight loss) plus:
   - a random plasma glucose concentration $\geq$ 11.1 mmol/L *or*
   - a fasting plasma glucose concentration $\geq$ 7.0 mmol/L (fasting is defined as no calorie intake for at least 8 hours) *or*
   - a 2 hour plasma glucose concentration $\geq$ 11.1 mmol/L during an oral glucose tolerance test (OGTT). OGTT is not recommended for routine clinical use.

2. With no symptoms, diagnosis should not be based on a single plasma glucose determination. At least one other plasma glucose on another day with a value in the diabetic range is essential, either fasting or at 120 min after a glucose load. If the fasting value is not diagnostic, the 120 min value should be used.

Impaired fasting glucose (IFG) and impaired glucose tolerance (IGT)

IFG: fasting plasma glucose $\geq$ 6.1 mmol/L but < 7.0 mmol/L.

IGT: fasting plasma glucose < 7.0 mmol/L and 2 hour plasma glucose during an OGTT $\geq$ 7.8 but < 11.1 mmol/L.

All subjects with IFG should have an oral glucose tolerance test (OGTT)

Gestational diabetes mellitus (GDM)

Gestational diabetes is defined as any degree of glucose intolerance with onset or first recognition during pregnancy. Strict glucose homeostasis is required during pregnancy in order to reduce the well-described diabetes-associated perinatal morbidity and mortality, as well as the associated maternal complications.

Although the majority of women who develop GDM return to normal after delivery, progression to overt diabetes often occurs in younger, thinner women. Other women have an increased risk of developing type 2 diabetes later in life. It is recommended that women with GDM are retested six weeks after delivery and classified as:

normal,
IFG (impaired fasting glucose),
IGT (impaired glucose tolerance),
diabetic.

Recommended targets for metabolic control in diabetes

	Good	Borderline	Poor
fasting plasma glucose (mmol/L)	4.4 - 6.1	6.2 - 7.8	> 7.8
post-prandial plasma glucose (mmol/L)	4.4 - 8.0	8.1 - 10.0	> 10.0
HbA1c (%)	< 6.5	6.5 - 7.5	> 7.5
urine glucose (%)	0	0 - 0.5	> 0.5
total cholesterol (mmol/L)	< 5.0	5.0 - 6.5	> 6.5
HDL cholesterol (mmol/L)	> 1.1	0.9 - 1.1	< 0.9
fasting triglyceride (mmol/L)	< 1.7	1.7 - 2.2	> 2.2
body mass index (kg/m^2) - Females	19 - 24	25 - 26	> 26
body mass index (kg/m^2) - Males	20 - 25	26 - 27	> 27
blood pressure (mm Hg)	< 135/85	135/85 - 160/90	>160/90
smoking	non-smoker	pipe	cigarettes

References

Alberti KGG, Gries FA, Jervell J, Kraqns HM. A desktop guide for the management of non-insulin-dependent diabetes mellitus (NIDDM): an update. European NIDDM Policy Group. Diab Med 1994; **11:** 899-909.

European Arterial Risk Policy Group on behalf of the International Diabetes Federation (European Region). A strategy for arterial risk assessment and management in type 2 (non-insulin-dependent) diabetes mellitus. Diab Med 1997; **14:** 611-21.

World Health Organisation. Definition, diagnosis and classification of diabetes mellitus and its complications. Geneva, 2000.

Hypoglycaemia

Acute hypoglycaemia may present with adrenergic symptoms, such as sweating, palpitation and tremor, or neuroglycopaenic symptoms such as cognitive impairment and ataxia. Symptoms occur with a plasma glucose less than 2.5 mmol/L and resolve on glucose administration. The commonest problem in evaluating such patients is that a blood sample is not taken at the time of hypoglycaemia for estimation of insulin and other analytes (see below). After excluding iatrogenic hypoglycaemia in patients with diabetes, the commonest cause of acute hypoglycaemia is alcohol intoxication.

More frequently patients present subacutely with episodes of cognitive impairment or presyncopal symptoms, which often resolve with carbohydrate ingestion. In these patients three 16 hour fasts are probably as effective at eliciting evidence of hypoglycaemia as the traditional 72 hour fast, using a blood glucose less than 3 mmol/L as diagnostic evidence and adding ketone body estimation to the diagnostic evaluation.

Reference
Marks V, Teale JD. Investigation of hypoglycaemia. Clin Endocrinol (Oxf) 1996; **44:** 133-6.

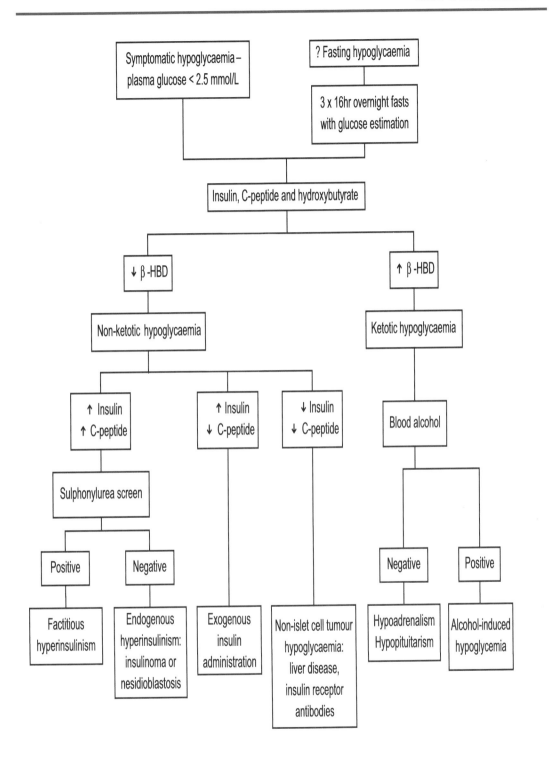

Polyuria

Polyuria is a subjective state although a daily loss of > 2.5 L urine with persistent urine osmolalities < 300 mmol/kg may be considered abnormal. The first line of investigation is to ascertain whether baseline values for urine volumes and plasma osmolality and sodium concentration are in fact abnormal. The next step is to determine if the increased urine production is driven by osmotically active substances excreted in the urine that cause obligate fluid loss e.g. glucose, ketones. It is then necessary to check if the water loss is due to either intrinsic tubular dysfunction or metabolic factors affecting tubular function e.g. hypokalaemia or hypercalcaemia. Polyuria is an infrequent manifestation of hyperthyroidism although a proportion of patients do complain of excessive thirst.

Often the most difficult patients to diagnose are those with psychogenic polydipsia. Many of these patients are investigated with water deprivation tests that are characterised by fluctuating urine volumes and osmolalities which mirror their surreptitious drinking during the test. It is important to exclude anticholinergic drugs that cause dryness of the mouth as a cause of increased fluid intake.

The hypertonic saline infusion test is included in this protocol for completeness. However, this is a potentially dangerous procedure and should probably only be performed in an experienced specialist unit.

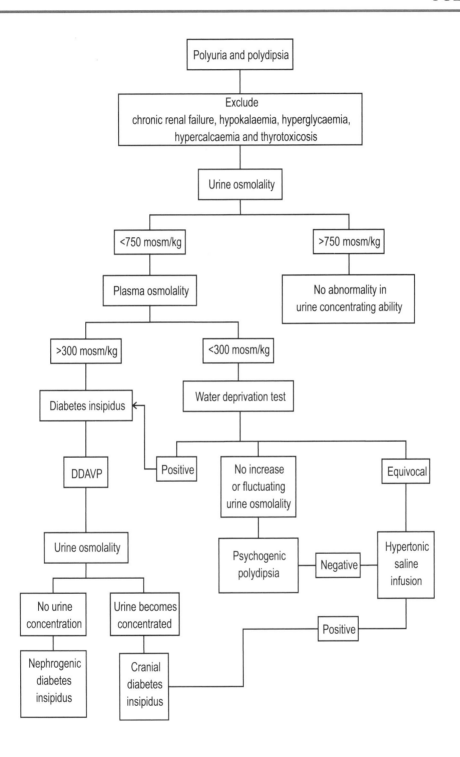

Hyponatraemia

Hyponatraemia may be either due to a deficiency of sodium or an excess of water. The determination of the hydration status of a patient is therefore the most important criterion in the evaluation of a hyponatraemic patient. Medical textbooks frequently cite reduced skin turgor, dry mouth and sunken eyeballs as signs of dehydration but these are only signs of severe dehydration. The use of haemodynamic variables e.g. pulse, arterial blood pressure and jugular (central) venous pressure give much earlier warning of fluid loss. The rate of urine flow is also a valuable sign but may be misleading in patients with renal disease or in states of osmotic diuresis.

Urine sodium is used as a critical step in this approach to hyponatraemia. However, sodium excretion as an obligate cation may occur even in hyponatraemic patients who are dehydrated with normal renal function. Examples include patients who become alkalotic with persistent vomiting and significant bicarbonaturia; or in patients with ketoacidosis who excrete large quantities of urinary ketoacids which have an effect as both osmotic diuretics and as anions requiring an obligate cation e.g. diabetic or alcoholic ketoacidosis or starvation.

Only in the acute presentation of adrenal failure is a high urinary sodium excretion consistently seen. In chronic cases, the reduced filtered load of sodium may lead to a new steady state with a lower urinary sodium concentration. Moreover, patients with pituitary disease and secondary adrenal failure may not be hypovolaemic due to the protective effect of ADH secretion.

Increased urinary sodium may occur in patients following subarachnoid haemorrhage or aneurysm surgery . This cerebral salt wasting may be due to excessive secretion of B type natriuretic peptide.

Acute versus chronic hyponatraemia

It is important to differentiate between acute and chronic hyponatraemia since the former has a mortality of up to 50%. Chronic hyponatraemia carries a better outcome but symptomatic cases have a mortality of 10 - 15%. Acute hyponatraemia may be defined as a plasma sodium concentration < 120 mmol/L developing over less than 48 hours or a fall in plasma sodium of greater than 0.5 mmol/h.

A recent analysis of hyponatraemia demonstrated a prevalence of 0.14% over a six month period in a district general hospital. After the exclusion of factitious causes, the majority of cases were due to chest infection, diuretics, cardiac failure, post-operative, other cases were related to malignancy and serotonin re-uptake inhibitors.

Syndrome of inappropriate ADH secretion (SIADH)

The diagnosis of SIADH is by exclusion and is based on the evaluation of a patient's hydration state, their general medical condition and presence of other diseases, drug therapy and the exclusion of endocrine causes of abnormalities of water homeostasis e.g. thyroid, pituitary and adrenal failure. SIADH is characterised by plasma hypotonicity with concentrated urine with high sodium excretion. Measurement of ADH is rarely required.

Cerebral salt wasting

Cerebral salt wasting is characterised by dehydration, hyponatraemia, massive urinary sodium loss and typically complicates cases of hypothalamic damage. Patients with subarachnoid haemorrhage have raised concentrations of the brain natriuretic peptide which appears to be raised in proportion to the intracranial pressure. This is associated with a suppression of the normal salt and water homeostatic mechanism: both plasma ADH and the renin-aldosterone axis are suppressed. The diagnosis should be considered in all cases of cerebral injury since plasma volume loss > 10% occurs in 50% of patients with subarachnoid haemorrhage.

References

Crook M, Velauthar U, Moran L, Griffiths W. The investigation and management of severe hyponatraemia in a hospital population. Ann Clin Biochem 1999; **36:** 158-62.

Harrigan MR. Cerebral salt wasting - a review. Neurosurgery 1996; **38:** 152-60.

Kumar S, Berl T. Sodium. Lancet 1998; **352:** 220-8.

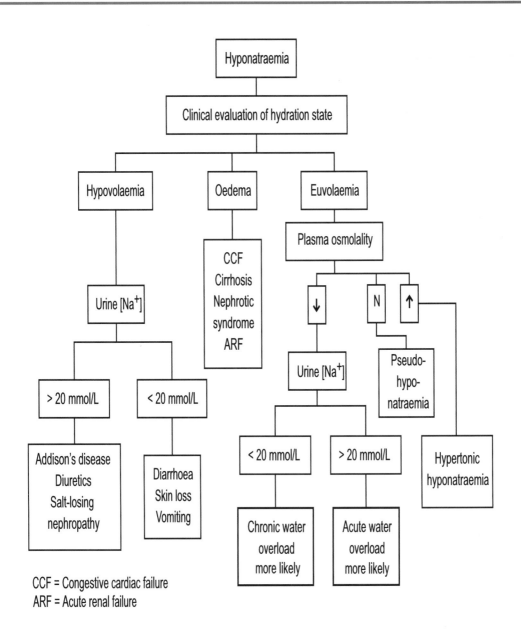

CCF = Congestive cardiac failure
ARF = Acute renal failure

Hypernatraemia

Hypernatraemia may be due to a failure of urine concentration by the kidneys. This results in the loss of hypotonic urine with the consequence that there is a rise in total body sodium which is reflected by hypernatraemia. Clinical evidence of dehydration may be evident in haemodynamic variables e.g. pulse, arterial blood pressure and jugular (central) venous pressure, and also a fall in urine output.

Most patients with hypernatraemia secondary to water loss do not appear dehydrated as water loss without sodium does not lead to overt volume contraction and the increased osmolality may be compensated by increased drinking (see polyuria)

Insensible losses are likely with febrile illnesses and hypermetabolic states associated with poor fluid intake.

Reference
Kumar S, Berl T. Sodium. Lancet 1998; **352:** 220-8.

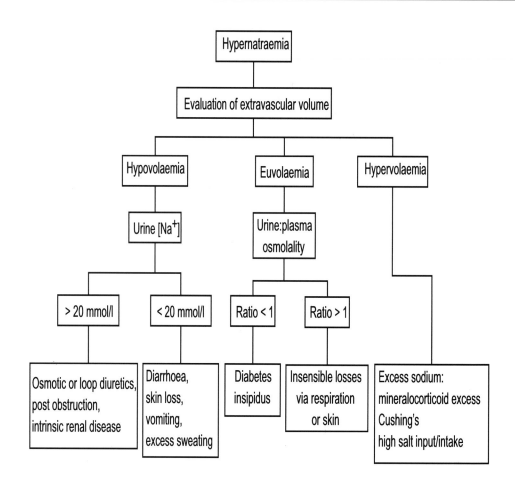

Hypokalaemia

Hypokalaemia is usually the result of potassium depletion due to renal or intestinal losses. Renal losses are most frequently due to metabolic alkalosis whereas intestinal losses are due to diarrhoea. Occasionally drugs are responsible for an acute shift from extra- to intra-cellular spaces, but this is rarely of clinical significance.

Intestinal potassium losses
Potassium loss in normal stools is very low. However, in diarrhoea the potassium concentration can be up to approximately 80-90 mmol/L.

Hypokalaemia in alkalosis
- This is most commonly due to vomiting. The mechanism is complex and is the result of a combination of factors including potassium loss in the vomitus (10 mmol/L) and urine, and an intracellular shift secondary to β-adrenergic stimulation. Overall fluid loss activates aldosterone secretion which enhances urine potassium loss.
- Excess mineralocorticoid action (primary or secondary).
- Genetic abnormalities of renal ion transporters.

Hypokalaemia in acidosis (rare)
- Type 1 renal tubular acidosis (see acidification protocols).
- In uncontrolled diabetes, especially diabetic ketoacidosis, the high urine glucose will cause an osmotic diuresis resulting in considerable sodium delivery to the distal tubules. This causes excessive urinary potassium loss which in the presence of relative haemoconcentration with elevated plasma potassium concentration may mask a reduced total body potassium. However, with treatment this potassium depletion will become apparent as hypokalaemia.

Oral potassium replacement
Ideally, potassium is replaced as the chloride salt (as in most therapeutic preparations) as most losses (e.g. as a result of diuretics, vomiting or nasogastric aspiration) are associated with chloride loss . Many fruits (e.g. figs, other dried fruits, nuts, avocados, bran cereals) have a high potassium content but these are phosphate salts and will need to be accompanied by sufficient chloride intake.

References
Gennari FJ. Hypokalaemia. New Engl J Med 1998; **339:** 451-8

Halperin ML, Kamel KS. Potassium. Lancet 1998; **352:** 135-40.

Cohn JN, Kowey PR, Whelton PK, Prisant LM. New guidelines for potassium replacement in clinical practice. Arch Intern Med 2000; **160:** 2429-36

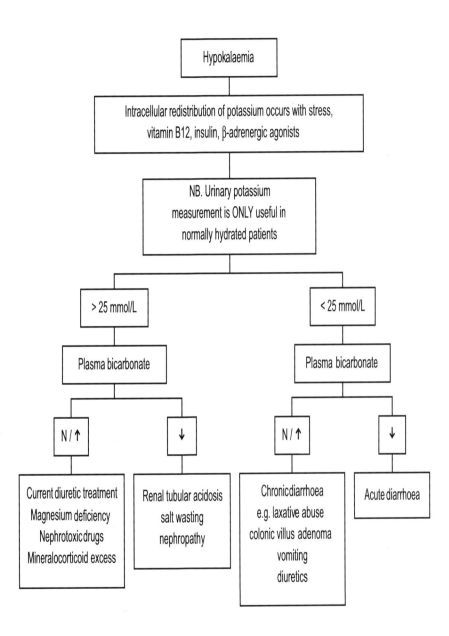

Hyperkalaemia

Factitious causes of hyperkalaemia

Mild hyperkalaemia due to factitious causes is almost impossible to exclude. Plasma potassium concentration rises in warm weather and with exercise; with delayed separation of plasma a rise in 1 mmol/L can occur in as little as four hours. In these cases, as well as those due to refrigeration, there will be no visible signs of haemolysis. Potassium concentration is slightly higher in serum than plasma due to release from leukocytes and platelets; this is only significant with marked leucocytosis (> 100×10^9/L) or thrombocytosis (> 400×10^9/L).

Tissue trauma

Intracellular potassium concentration is approximately 100 mmol/L and only small shifts are required to raise plasma concentrations. The commonest cause of release of intracellular potassium release is haemolysis but other causes include trauma, rhabdomyolysis and cell lysis with cancer chemotherapy.

Drugs that may cause hyperkalaemia
digoxin (toxic concentrations)
succinylcholine
heparin
ACE inhibitors
NSAIDs (occasionally)
drugs decreasing distal tubular secretion of potassium: amiloride, spironolactone, triamterene

Reference

Halperin ML, Kamel KS. Potassium. Lancet 1998; **352:** 135-40.

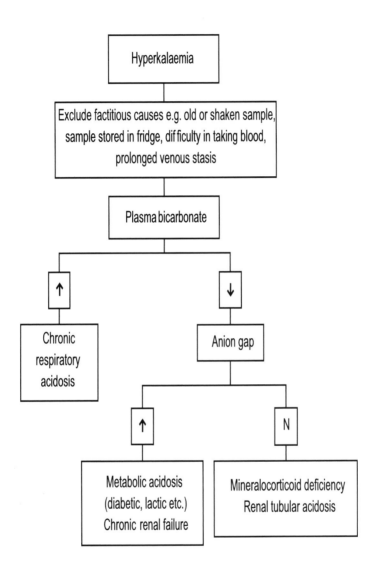

Hypocalcaemia

In hospital practice, hypocalcaemia is most commonly seen in subjects with dietary vitamin D deficiency or as a transient event after total thyroidectomy. Hypoparathyroidism is most commonly due to surgical removal but may also be caused by autoimmunity, infiltration by amyloid or heavy metals e.g. iron in haemochromatosis or thalassaemia, or copper in Wilson's disease.

Hypocalcaemia can occur in acute pancreatitis, largely as a result of the release of pancreatic lipase into the retroperitoneal space and peritoneal cavity, where it saponifies fat, releasing free fatty acids which bind calcium. Hypocalcaemia in pancreatitis is associated with a poor prognosis. The fall in calcium is usually gradual and investigation for the cause should be delayed until the pancreatitis has settled. This is to ensure that any changes in PTH are not secondary to changes in the plasma calcium. Treatment for hypocalcaemia is probably only necessary if symptoms e.g. cramps or parasthesiae occur. The mechanism for hypocalcaemia in endotoxic shock is currently unknown.

Hyperventilation, for example in acute anxiety states or head injury, causes an acute respiratory alkalosis. This allows increased binding of calcium to plasma proteins so that symptoms of hypocalcaemia may occur because of reduced ionised calcium though the total calcium concentration is normal.

Abnormally low plasma concentrations of magnesium, phosphate and potassium are frequently (20-30%) detected in association with hypocalcaemia and these abnormalities should be corrected as they may be the primary cause or, at least, an exacerbating factor of the hypocalcaemia due to their effects on renal tubular function and, in the case of magnesium, on the inhibition of PTH synthesis and secretion.

Reference
Bushinsky DA, Monk RD. Calcium. Lancet 1998; **352:** 306-11.

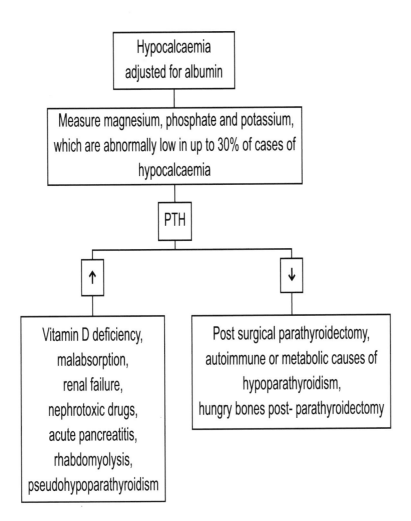

Hypercalcaemia

The albumin bound fraction of calcium accounts for approximately half plasma calcium and is physiologically inactive. Ideally, ionised calcium should be measured but available techniques are not suitable for routine use. An adjustment for the effect of abnormal concentrations of albumin may therefore be made to help interpret total plasma calcium estimations. The precise formula for calcium adjustment will depend on laboratory methods and should be derived locally.

The commonest cause of hypercalcaemia in the community is a parathyroid adenoma although in hospital practice excess therapeutic vitamin D (or vitamin D derivatives) and malignancy are more frequent. It is important to note that 10-15% of cases of hypercalcaemia associated with malignancy also have hyperparathyroidism. This subgroup should be identified as these individuals have considerably longer rates of survival than those with purely malignancy-associated hypercalcaemia.

Effect of drug therapies

Many patients with hypercalcaemia will be dehydrated on presentation and should be adequately rehydrated before investigation. Samples for PTH, etc. MUST be taken before any other active treatment. This is because bisphosphonates cause a rapid increase in PTH as a consequence of the fall in calcium, even before the plasma calcium has fallen into the reference range.

The hypercalcaemia of vitamin D intoxication may last for many weeks after cessation of vitamin D intake since 25-OHvitamin D has a long elimination half life (10-20 days).

Hypercalcaemia revealed by thiazide diuretics may be due to volume contraction with an increase in calcium binding proteins but can also be due to increased renal tubular absorption of calcium. Thiazide treatment may unmask patients with early hyperparathyroidism or vitamin D excess.

Familial hypocalciuric hypercalcaemia (FHH)

FHH is an inherited condition in which the plasma calcium is 'set' at a high value. Affected individuals do not suffer from any of the complications of hypercalcaemia and parathyroidectomy has no effect of plasma calcium. The diagnosis can be made by measuring urine calcium excretion, which is lower than would be expected in the hypercalcaemia of hyperparathyroidism. PTH is often marginally raised in FHH despite mild hypercalcaemia and it is important that FHH is considered in the differential diagnosis

FHH is defined by the following biochemical criteria:

- 24h urine calcium < 6.25 mmol in presence of raised plasma calcium

- calcium:creatinine molar ratio < 0.01

- fasting calcium excretion rate < 22 μmol/L glomerular filtration in presence of raised plasma calcium and detectable PTH.

References

Barth JH, Fiddy JB, Payne RB. Adjustment of serum total calcium for albumin concentration: effects of non-linearity and regression differences between laboratories. Ann Clin Biochem 1996; **33:** 55-8.

Gunn IR, Wallace JR. Urine calcium and serum ionized calcium, total calcium and parathyroid hormone concentrations in the diagnosis of primary hyperparathyroidism and familial benign hypercalcaemia. Ann Clin Biochem 1992; **29:** 52-8.

Hutchesson AC, Bundred NJ, Ratcliffe WA. Survival in hypercalcaemic patients with cancer and co-existing hyperparathyroidism. Postgrad Med J 1995; **71:** 28-31.

Marx SJ, Attie MF, Levine MA, Spiegel AM, Downs RW Jr, Lasker RD. The hypocalciuric or benign variant of familial hypercalcaemia: clinical and biochemical features in fifteen kindreds. Medicine 1981; **60:** 397-412.

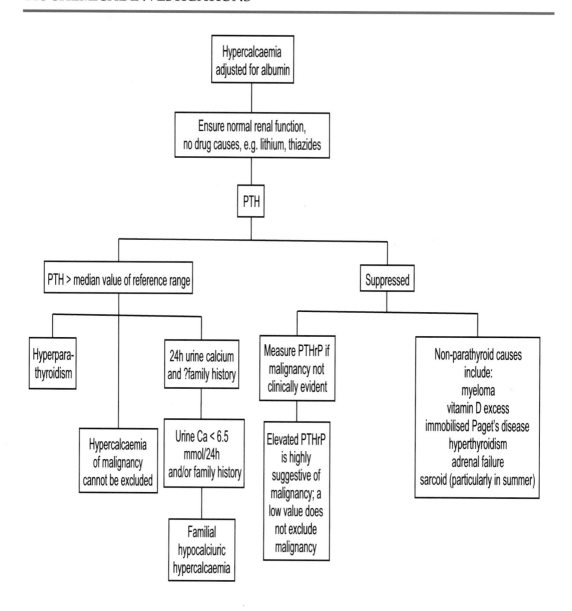

Hypophosphataemia

Hypophosphataemia (less than 0.7 mmol/L) occurs in as many as 25% of hospital inpatients. However, functional deficiency does not occur until plasma phosphate falls below 0.3 mmol/L. At this concentration, replacement should be considered urgently since severe hypophosphataemia usually indicates insufficient intracellular phosphate, limiting ATP synthesis and can result in widespread organ failure.

The features of phosphate deficiency include haemolysis, thrombocytopenia and poor granulocyte function. Severe muscle weakness, respiratory muscle failure and rhabdomyolysis can occur. Confusion, irritability and coma may be due to a metabolic encephalopathy caused by phosphate deficiency.

The first diagnostic step is to determine whether hypophosphataemia is due to real deficiency or due to redistribution within the body since the latter is benign. However, in all but short term cases of hypophosphataemia, redistribution is also associated with the conditions that cause renal phosphate loss. Therefore, a pragmatic approach is to consider that individuals with moderately low plasma phosphate (0.48-0.72 mmol/L) do not need replacement unless they have a risk factor for phosphate depletion, whereas if the plasma phosphate is below 0.32 mmol/L, phosphate depletion is likely and replacement should be administered.

References

Crook M, Swaminathan R. Disorders of plasma phosphate and indications for its measurement. Ann Clin Biochem 1996; **33:** 376-96.

Payne RB. Renal tubular reabsorption of phosphate (TmP/GFR): indications and interpretation. Ann Clin Biochem 1998; **35:** 201-6.

Weisinger JR, Bellorin-Font E. Magnesium and phosphorus. Lancet 1998; **352:** 391-396.

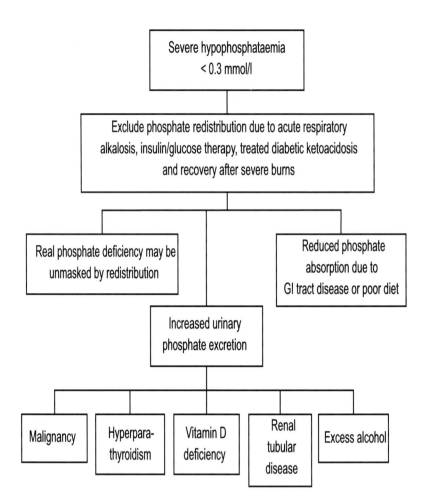

Hyperphosphataemia

Renal failure is the commonest cause of hyperphosphataemia in clinical practice.

Spurious elevations in phosphate occur with paraproteinaemia, hyperlipidaemia, haemolysis and hyperbilirubinaemia and these should be considered in unexplained hyperphosphataemia.

Hyperphosphataemia is common in lactic acidosis and may reflect loss of intracellular phosphate following hydrolysis of ATP.

Hyperphosphatemia often occurs in patients receiving phosphate enemas.

Rapid elevations in phosphate may result in hypocalcaemia and precipitation of calcium phosphate crystals (metastatic calcification). Although hypocalcaemia is the usual response to raised phosphate, if the latter is caused by bone breakdown, then elevations in both calcium and phosphate may ensue.

Symptoms and signs of hyperphosphataemia	
Heart	conduction disturbances, heart failure
Kidneys	oliguria
GI tract	anorexia, nausea, vomiting, ileus, GI bleeding
Lungs	breathlessness, reduced oxygen diffusion
Eyes	conjunctival inflammation
Skin	papules, digital ischaemia

Reference
Weisinger JR, Bellorin-Font E. Magnesium and phosphorus. Lancet 1998; **352:** 391-6.

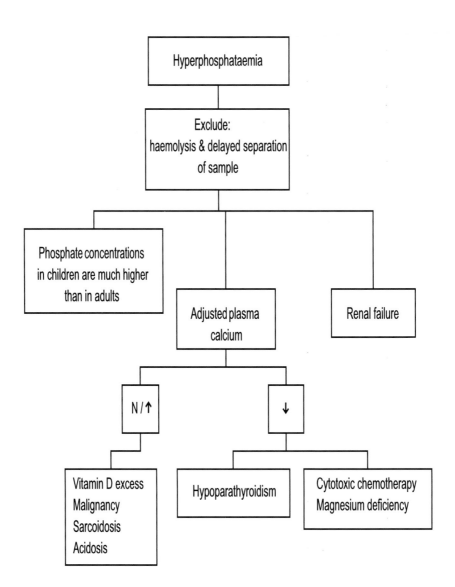

Investigation of renal stones

All patients presenting acutely with renal stones should have measurements of plasma creatinine, calcium and urate. The importance of knowing their renal function is to determine the urgency with which further investigations and treatment should be performed so that further renal damage can be avoided. Other investigations will include imaging of the renal tract and urine culture (including examination for fastidious organisms). This diagnostic algorithm is designed for the investigation of patients following their acute presentation.

Renal stones will occur in 8-15% of Europeans and North Americans during their lives. The majority of stones (~ 80%) are composed of calcium phosphate and most of the remainder are composed of uric acid (5-10%), struvite or carbonate apatite (secondary to infection) or cystine (~ 1%). Stones composed of other compounds occur rarely.

Investigation of the aetiology of renal stones is based on urine chemistry rather than analysis of the stone itself because the accuracy of stone analysis is generally poor and, even when accurate, does not explain the pathophysiology of stone formation except in the rare inherited disorders e.g. cystinuria.

The rationale of not investigating those patients with a single stone and no risk factors is largely arbitrary since approximately 75% of patients presenting with a renal stone will have a recurrence during the next 20 years. The decision about the degree of investigation and the potential for life long therapies will depend on the patient.

The presence of diseases of the chest and GI tract and some drugs are important insofar as they affect the excretion of acid in the urine (see below).

The importance of measuring urine pH

Urine pH should be measured on fresh urine samples as urine is not strongly buffered and carbon dioxide will evaporate. The inability to acidify urine during an episode of acidosis (either spontaneous or therapeutically induced) indicates a form of renal tubular acidosis and a direct tubular effect on calcium excretion. However, the main reason for measuring urine pH, since few patients with renal stones will have RTA, is to determine if stone formation is secondary to subtle changes in urinary pH. This may reduce the solubility of supersaturated salts in urine and enhance crystal formation. In view of this we would suggest that normal urine has a pH range of 6-7 and that it may be appropriate to consider therapies to alter urine pH in recurrent stone formers whose urine pH is outside these limits.

Urinary urea is measured to give a guide to protein intake for the evaluation of urate (i.e. purine) excretion.

24 hours urine volumes

It is important to record measurement of the total urine volume passed over each of the 24 hour collections since poor urine flow effectively increases the concentration of salts and will enhance crystal formation.

Hypertension

Hypertension is considered a risk factor since there is a strong association between the two conditions with a suggestion that hypertension develops after the presentation of stones. Moreover, hypertensive patients have a considerably higher degree of calciuria than controls.

Renal stones in children

This algorithm is not suitable for children with renal stones because children are more likely to have renal stones related to inborn errors of metabolism.

References

Coe FL, Parks JH, Asplin JR. The pathogenesis and treatment of kidney stones. New Eng J Med 1992; **327:** 1141-52.

Madore F, Stampfer MJ, Rimm EB, Curhan GC. Nephrolithiasis and risk of hypertension. Am J Hypertens 1998; **11:** 46-53.

Pak CYC. Kidney stones. Lancet 1998; **351:** 1797-800.

Quereda C, Orte L, Sabater J, Navarro-Antolin J, Villafruela JJ, Ortuna J. Urinary calcium excretion in treated and untreated essential hypertension. J Am Soc Nephrol 1996; **7:** 1058-65.

Wilkinson H. Clinical investigation and management of patients with renal stones. Ann Clin Biochem 2001; **38:** 180-7.

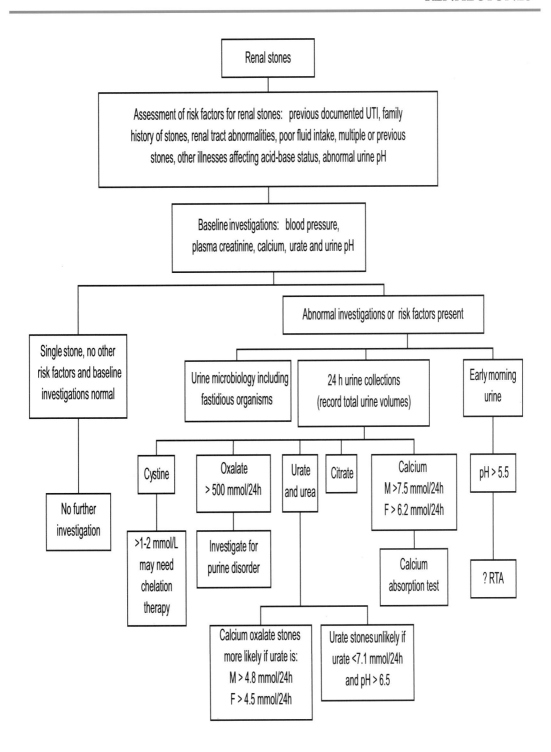

Effect of renal failure on hormones

Pathophysiological mechanisms on endocrine function
- Increased concentration of hormones or hormone fragments
  - impaired degradation e.g. insulin, PTH, calcitonin
  - increased secretion e.g. insulin, PTH

- Decreased concentration due to reduced production
  - renal hormones e.g. erythropoetin, 1,25-OHvitamin D3
  - extrarenal hormones e.g. oestradiol, testosterone

- Disturbances of hormone action
  - disturbed prohormone activation e.g. T4 to T3
  - multimolecular forms e.g. glycosylation isoforms e.g. LH
  - altered binding to carrier proteins e.g. somatomedins
  - altered target organ sensitivity e.g. GH, insulin

Thyroid function in chronic renal failure (CRF)
Approximately 50% euthyroid patients with CRF have an enlarged thyroid gland if not a palpable goitre. The prevalence of hypothyroidism varies between studies at 0-9.5%. This increased (2.5 fold) prevalence matches an increase in the finding of thyroid peroxidase antibodies.

Thyroid function tests in CRF
- TSH not affected and is probably the best guide of thyroid status.

- Total T4 and T3 are often low especially when GFR < 50%.

- Thyroid hormones bind to pre-albumin, albumin and TBG. Plasma concentrations of these proteins are usually normal in patients on haemodialysis but low in those on CAPD probably due to peritoneal protein loss.

- Analytical differences: by equilibrium dialysis fT4 and fT3 may be normal or high, whereas direct assays of total or free hormones tend to give low values.

- TRH testing shows a blunted but prolonged TSH response, probably due to delayed clearance of TSH and TRH.

- Overall there is experimental data to suggest interference with all levels of the hypothalamo-pituitary-thyroid axis with an alteration of the 'thyrostat'.

Pituitary-adrenal axis in CRF

Clinical features of excess cortisol (osteopenia, proximal myopathy, hypertension and glucose intolerance) and reduced cortisol (hypotension, weakness and hypokalaemia) can also be features of chronic renal failure and the diagnosis of Cushing's syndrome or adrenal insufficiency depends on biochemical tests.

Conventional Synacthen (ACTH) tests give normal cortisol responses.

Uraemic patients may show sub-optimal plasma cortisol suppression after oral dexamethasone. It is unknown if this is due to poor intestinal absorption of dexamethasone or increased plasma clearance.

References

Ramirez G, Gomez-Sanchez C, Meikle WA, Jubiz W. Evaluation of the hypothalamic hypophyseal adrenal axis in patients receiving long-term dialysis. Arch Intern Med 1982; **142:** 1448-52.

Ramirez G, Brueggemeyer C, Ganguly A. Counterregulatory hormone responses to insulin-induced hypoglycaemia in patients on chronic hemodialysis. Nephron 1988; **49:** 231-6.

Renal tubular acidosis

Introduction

Acid excretion is one of the main roles of the kidney; congenital and acquired disorders of the nephron result in acidosis. Whilst chronic renal failure remains the commonest form of acidosis, isolated tubular defects represent a more challenging diagnostic dilemma. The inherited forms are characterised by a hyperchloraemic acidosis with near normal GFR and plasma inorganic anions e.g. phosphate.

	Classic distal RTA (Type I)	Incomplete distal RTA (Type II)	Voltage dependent distal RTA (Type I)	Proximal RTA (Type II)	Type IV RTA
Urine pH*	>5.5	>5.5	>5.5	<5.5	<5.5
Urine anion gap*	Positive	Negative	Positive	Negative	Positive
Fractional bicarbonate excretion**	< 5 - 10%	< 5 - 10%	< 5 - 10%	> 15%	5 - 15%
Frusemide test	Abnormal	Abnormal	Abnormal (if reversible)	Normal	Normal
Urine calcium*	High	Normal/ high	High	Normal	Normal
Urine citrate*	Low	Low/ normal	Low	Normal	Normal
Renal stones	Common	Common	Common	Rare	Rare
Metabolic bone disease	Rare	Rare	Rare	Common	Rare
Other tubular defects	Rare	Rare	Rare	Common	Rare
Plasma potassium*	Normal/ low	Normal	High	Normal/ low	High

*   determined when plasma bicarbonate < 20 mmol/L
**   determined when plasma bicarbonate > 26 mmol/L

Urine pH

The ideal sample for measuring pH is a fresh early morning urine taken before breakfast. It is important to be certain that the urine is sterile as urea splitting organisms release ammonia and increase the pH.

Urine anion gap (UAG)

This is an indirect method for measuring urine [ammonia] and can be measured on a random urine sample. It is only valid when the urine pH < 6.5 as at greater pH, urine bicarbonate is a significant anion.

$$UAG = (urine\ [Na^+] + urine\ [K^+]) - urine\ [Cl^-]$$

The use of the UAG as an estimate of urine ammonium ion is disputed by some investigators.

Fractional bicarbonate excretion (FE (HCO$_3^-$))

FE can be assessed on a random urine sample. Take care to ensure that the sample container is full and there is a minimum air space available for loss of bicarbonate by evaporation. NB: ensure that creatinine and bicarbonate results are in the same units.

$$FE\ (HCO_3^-) = (plasma\ HCO_3^-\ x\ urine\ creatinine)/(plasma\ creatinine\ x\ urine\ HCO_3^-)$$

Hypokalaemia

Hypokalamia or chronic acidosis may prevent normal urinary acidification and urine pH will be > 5.5, due to increased tubular ammoniagenesis. Hyponatraemia may also prevent acidification due to reduced cation available for exchange in the distal tubules.

Reference ranges for urinary analytes

Random urine citrate (adults) 1.6-4.5 mmol/24 hours or > 100 µmol/mmol creatinine, (children) > 75 (males) > 177 (females) µmol/mmol creatinine.
Urine ammonia (adults) 36-99 µmol/min/1.73 m^2, , (children under 15 years) 49-119 µmol/min/1.73 m^2

Reference

Kirschbaum B, Sica D, Anderson P. Urine electrolytes and the urine anion and osmolar gaps. J Lab Clin Med 1999; **133:** 597-604.

Penney MD, Oleesky DA. Renal tubular acidosis. Ann Clin Biochem 1999; **36:** 408-22.

Confusion

The first step in the differential diagnosis of a confused patient is to determine whether it is due to primary neurological disease or a manifestation of a systemic disorder. Localising neurological signs are generally a sign of neurological disease but may be induced by hypoglycaemia, especially in the elderly. Infection should be considered even in the absence of fever and chest X-ray, blood and urine cultures performed. The choice of investigations will be governed by the clinical history and signs.

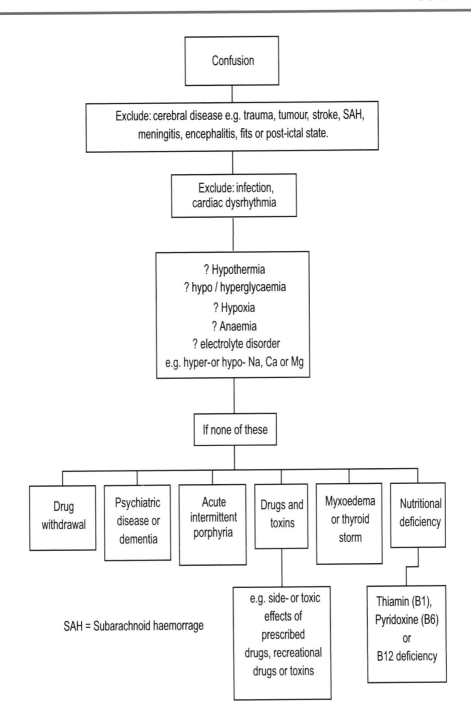

Confusion

Exclude: cerebral disease e.g. trauma, tumour, stroke, SAH, meningitis, encephalitis, fits or post-ictal state.

Exclude: infection, cardiac dysrhythmia

? Hypothermia
? hypo / hyperglycaemia
? Hypoxia
? Anaemia
? electrolyte disorder
e.g. hyper- or hypo- Na, Ca or Mg

If none of these

Drug withdrawal

Psychiatric disease or dementia

Acute intermittent porphyria

Drugs and toxins

Myxoedema or thyroid storm

Nutritional deficiency

e.g. side- or toxic effects of prescribed drugs, recreational drugs or toxins

Thiamin (B1), Pyridoxine (B6) or B12 deficiency

SAH = Subarachnoid haemorrage

Excessive generalised sweating

Generalised sweating is usually thermoregulatory, emotional (stress) or gustatory. Thermoregulatory sweating is generally worse during sleep as is the form associated with systemic illness. Gustatory sweating is usually localised to the face but more generalised involvement may be a feature of generalised sympathetic nervous system disorders. It is quite common after surgery to the parotid gland.

Generalised increase in sweating may be a feature of endocrinopathies e.g. acromegaly, carcinoid or diabetes, but is rarely a diagnostic problem. Very obese patients also complain of excessive sweating but this is usually in response to unaccustomed exercise.

Asymmetrical sweating may be due to localised skin disorders or disorders of the sympathetic nervous system but it is rare for sweating to be the only clinical feature.

Drugs recognised to cause sweating
anticholinesterases chlorpropamide (with alcohol) corticosteroids danazol fluoxetine moclobemide opiates pilocarpine tricyclic antidepressants venlafaxine

References

Davies DM (ed). Textbook of adverse drug reactions. Oxford: Oxford University Press. 4th edit 1991.

Gelman Gr, Rumack BH (eds). Drugdex® Information System. Denver: Micromedex Inc.

Sato K, Kang WH, Saga K, Sato KT. Biology of sweat glands and their disorders.II. Disorders of sweat gland function. J Am Acad Dermatol 1989; **20:** 713-26.

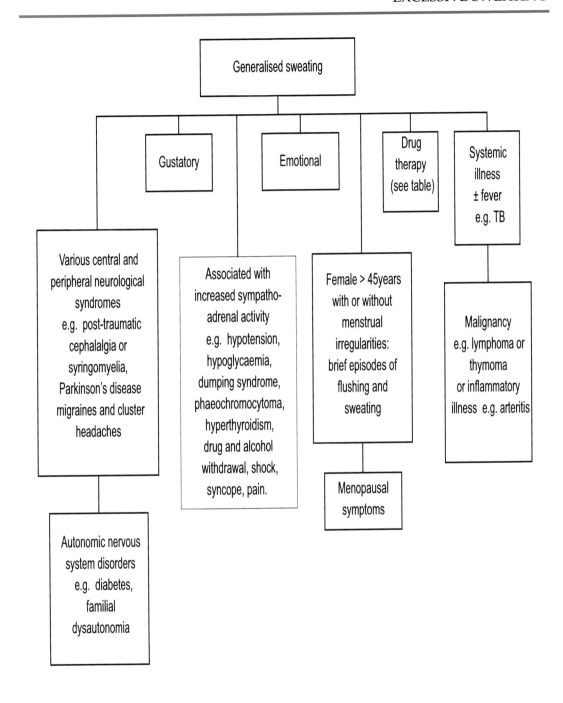

Flushing

Flushing is a well recognised phenomenon of transient cutaneous vasodilatation caused by emotional, autonomic or endocrine influences, or pharmacological factors. Menopausal flushing may develop in the male after orchidectomy or GnRH therapy for prostate cancer. Histamine flushes may be due to large quantities of histamine in some alcoholic beverages, to the pharmacological effect of some drugs, or mast cell disease. Flushing often occurs in anaphylactic reactions but it is invariably associated with other systemic symptoms e.g. urticaria, upper airway obstruction, etc. Alcohol may induce flushing even without chlorpropamide, metronidazole or disulfiram.

Idiopathic flushing

Flushing is more likely to be idiopathic in young female patients than due to carcinoid. Features characteristic of idiopathic flushing include palpitations, syncope and hypotensive episodes whereas carcinoid is more likely to cause wheezing and abdominal pain. Diarrhoea occurs in both conditions.

Recurrent unexplained flushing

This disorder has been described in ten patients. Patients reported attacks of flushing lasting 15 minutes to 2 days and associated with such symptoms as anxiety, chest tightness, parasthesia, slurred speech, weakness and pruritus. Abdominal pain was a constant feature, often associated with cramping and an increase in stool frequency. Attacks witnessed by physicians consisted of an exaggerated blush response of the face and upper part of the chest, and were sometimes associated with tachycardia, mild hypertension, and tachypnoea. Urticaria, angioedema, wheezing, and hypotension were not observed. This condition is characterised by repeatedly negative investigations performed over many years.

Drugs recognised to cause flushing	
antidepressants	levodopa
amyl nitrite	metronidazole (with alcohol)
β-blockers	nicotinic acid
calcium channel blockers	nitrates
cephalosporins (with alcohol)	oxybutynin
chlorpropamide (with alcohol)	pilocarpine
danazol	tretinoin
desmopressin	TRH
histamine	

References

Aldrich LB, Moattari AR, Vinik AI. Distinguishing features of idiopathic flushing and carcinoid syndrome. Arch Intern Med 1988; **148:** 2614-8.

Davies DM (ed). Textbook of adverse drug reactions. Oxford: Oxford University Press. 4th ed. 1991.

Friedman BS, Germano P, Miletti J, Metcalfe DD. A clinicopathologic study of ten patients with recurrent unexplained flushing. J Allergy Clin Immunol 1994; **93:** 53-8.

Gelman Gr, Rumack BH (eds). Drugdex® Information System. Denver: Micromedex Inc.

Winbury SL, Lieberman PL. Anaphylaxis. Immunol Allergy Clin NA 1995; **15:** 447-75.

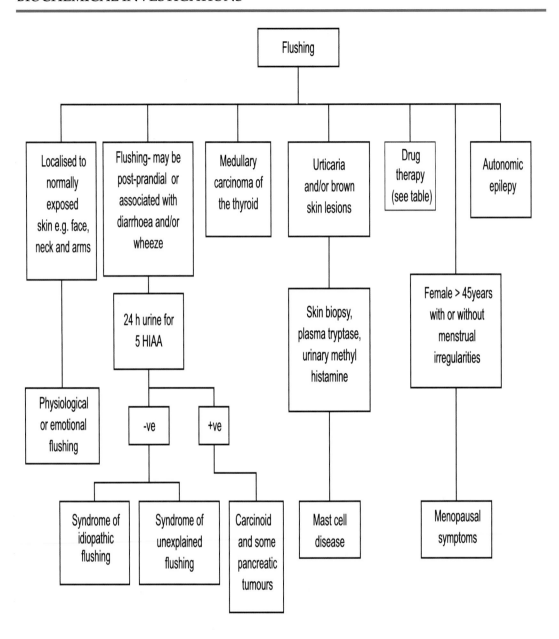

Generalised itching

Patients with scratch marks but without a recognisable dermatosis may have an underlying metabolic abnormality. There are a large number of causes and the nature and sequence of investigations will depend on the history and clinical signs.

Dermatological disorders

Skin disorders are the most frequent cause of itching and can usually be diagnosed by their appearance. However, it is important to recognise that scratch marks and secondary dermatoses can be due to non-dermatological conditions.

Metabolic disorders

Obstructive biliary disease e.g. primary biliary cirrhosis, pregnancy-associated
  cholestasis
Renal failure
Haematological disorders e.g. polycythaemia rubra vera, iron deficiency, mastocy-
  tosis
Thyroid disease
CNS disorders
Lymphoma
Other/malignancy

The best investigation for pruritus thought to be caused by malignancy is a thorough clinical examination.

Drugs

Associated with cholestasis	Others
anabolic steroids	aspirin
chlopromazine	chloroquine
erythromycin	canthaxanthin
phenothiazines	carbamazepine
tolbutamide	cromoglycate
	dexamethasone, hydrocortisone
	gold salts
	invermectin
	isoniazid
	opiates
	quinidine
	streptomycin

Pregnancy

Intrahepatic cholestasis of pregnancy produces generalised itching which may or may not eventually be accompanied by jaundice. It may begin as early as the twentieth week of pregnancy and remits promptly after delivery. LFTs reveal increased bilirubin and alkaline phosphatase with normal transaminases.

AIDS

Patients with AIDS may have primary pruritus but it is usually due to an inflammatory or infective dermatosis.

Reference

Gelman GR, Rumack BH (eds). Drugdex® Information System. Denver: Micromedex Inc.

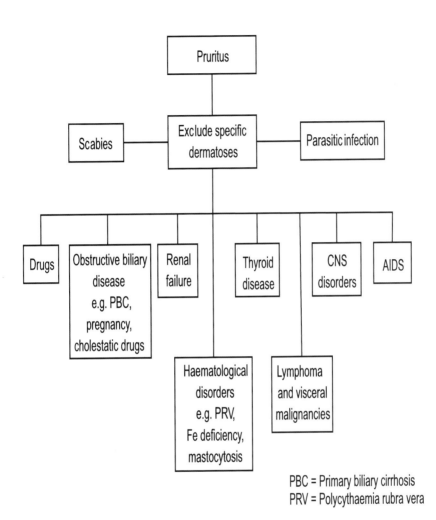

PBC = Primary biliary cirrhosis
PRV = Polycythaemia rubra vera

Hereditary haemochromatosis (HH)

Haemochromatosis is an inherited condition in which too much iron is absorbed from the diet. Iron accumulation in many organs causes the clinical manifestations, which include diabetes and cirrhosis of the liver. Clinical problems are usually seen in middle age but sometimes occur in people as young as 20 years. Haemochromatosis is inherited as an autosomal recessive disorder. Treatment involves removing the excess iron by weekly venesections for up to two years. If the diagnosis is made before the development of cirrhosis of the liver, iron removal usually prevents the clinical problems and restores normal life expectancy.

Clinical features of haemochromatosis

In early disease there may be no diagnostic features. However, many tissues are affected by iron deposition which results in skin pigmentation, diabetes mellitus, liver and cardiac disease, arthropathy and primary and secondary hypogonadism.

Diagnosis of iron overload

The diagnosis of haemochromatosis is suggested by the demonstration of transferrin saturation > 55% (men) or > 50% (women) in a fasting sample (transferrin saturation = (Fe/TIBC) x 100%). A diagnosis of haemochromatosis is only made in a proportion of subjects with raised non-fasting transferrin saturation. Ferritin concentration is usually elevated, particularly in the presence of liver disease, but may be normal in the early stages of iron accumulation. Confirmation may be made by liver biopsy.

Following the demonstration of iron overload, secondary causes of iron overload need to be excluded before haemochromatosis can be diagnosed. These include porphyria cutanea tarda, beta thalassaemia intermedia, hereditary spherocytosis and sideroblastic anaemia. False positive raised transferrin saturation may occur in patients with fatty liver, alcoholic liver disease and haematological conditions.

Liver iron determination

Liver biopsies (3 - 10 mg wet weight) should be transferred to the laboratory in dry containers as quickly as possible for accurate measurement of weight. Hepatic iron is classified by the hepatic iron index (Fe µmol/g dry weight divided by the age in years - normal < 1.9). Liver biopsy is not necessary for the diagnosis if mutations in the HFE gene are demonstrable, but may be useful to assess hepatic fibrosis.

Monitoring efficacy of venesection

Venesection should be performed sufficiently frequently to maintain plasma transferrin saturation below 60% and the ferritin concentration below 100 µg/L.

Genetic tests for the proband and family members

In the UK 90% of patients are homozygous for the Cys282Tyr mutation in the HFE gene. This mutation is present in approximately 1:250 of the UK population and its analysis, together with iron studies, can be used for screening families where a proband has been identified. It is unknown how many subjects homozygous for the Cys282Tyr mutation will eventually develop clinical haemochromatosis.

References

Niederau C, Fischer R, Purschel A, Stremmel W, Haussinger D, Strohmeyer G. Long term survival in patients with hereditary haemochromatosis. Gastroenterol 1996; **110:** 1107-19.

Dooley J, Worwood M. Genetic haemochromatosis. British Committee for Standards in Haematology. British Committee for Standards in Haematology. Darwin Medical Communications, Oxford. 2000.

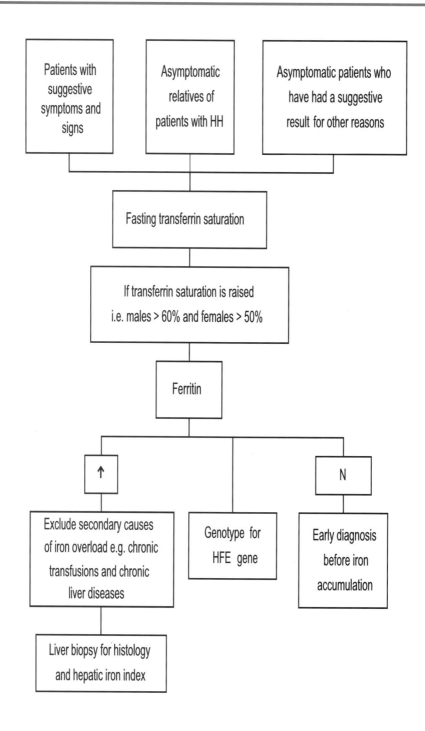

Hyperlipidaemia

Hyperlipidaemia is defined as an increase in the concentrations of cholesterol, triglycerides or both. 'Normal values' traditionally defined as 95% population ranges are not appropriate nowadays since so many people in developed, and, increasingly in developing, populations are at risk of ischaemic heart disease. Reference values are therefore replaced by decision points for treating patients with, or at risk, of ischaemic heart disease. Patients with hypercholesterolaemia need to be investigated to determine whether they need specific treatment to prevent IHD and/or their families need to be studied.

One of the most difficult aspects of the diagnosis of hyperlipidaemia is the lack of conclusive diagnostic tests for most of the disorders. This is particularly important for the different forms of isolated hypercholesterolaemia, and to distinguish familial combined hyperlipidaemia from other causes of mild hypertriglyceridaemia (i.e. approximately 2.5-6 mmol/L). Patients with hypertriglyceridaemia are more likely to have a secondary cause. However, it is important to recognise the primary cases since there is an increased risk of acute pancreatitis in individuals with very high concentrations of triglycerides.

Effect of acute illness of lipids
An acute event e.g. myocardial infarction or stroke, has a profound effect on circulating lipids causing a 30% fall in total cholesterol and 50% rise in triglycerides. These effects are maximal at seven days and take approximately three months to resolve.

When are HDL-cholesterol and LDL-cholesterol subfractions useful?
The importance of lipoprotein analysis is in the evaluation of risk for individuals assessed for primary or secondary prevention of IHD. Patients with proven IHD should be given lipid lowering therapy with the aim of maintaining total cholesterol < 5.0 mmol/L (or LDL-cholesterol < 3.0 mmol/L). All patients starting lipid lowering therapy should have a full lipid profile to ensure that the excess total cholesterol is due to LDL-cholesterol and not HDL-cholesterol or triglyceride-rich particles. This is particularly relevant for women who may retain a high HDL-cholesterol for many years after the menopause.

Lp(a)
Lipoprotein (a) is pro-atherogenic lipoprotein with a structure similar to plasminogen and which binds to LDL-cholesterol. It is associated with an increased risk of IHD. However, assays for it is are not routinely available since it is unstable in plasma and therefore not suitable for routine measurement. Furthermore, there are currently no therapies that reliably reduce Lp(a).

Primary hypertriglyceridaemia

The causes of primary hypertriglyceridaemia are relatively rare and need to be diagnosed biochemically since eruptive xanthomata can occur with hypertriglyceridaemia of any cause. The differential diagnosis is (i) remnant removal disease (familial dysbetalipoproteinaemia) (usually but not always associated with the apo-E genotype E2:E2); (ii) lipoprotein lipase (or its co-factor CII) deficiency, and (iii) familial hypertriglyceridaemia. The diagnosis of lipoprotein lipase deficiency is made on the basis of a failure of plasma lipase to rise after administration of IV heparin (exact protocol should be requested from the specialist laboratory performing this test); patients should have fasted overnight, refrained from alcohol for 24 hours and heavy exercise for 48 hours. The diagnosis of familial hypertriglyceridaemia is based on family studies and exclusion of the above disorders.

Random or fasting samples ?

The diagnosis of lipid abnormalities requires analysis of samples taken after 12 to 14 hour fast. However, since triglyceride concentrations rise by 200-300% after a meal, it is often useful to use random samples for screening since any abnormality in triglyceride pathways will be stressed and become apparent. There are minimal changes in total cholesterol and HDL-cholesterol in relation to meals although long term changes in diet will raise or lower triglycerides.

Reference

Joint recommendations on prevention of coronary heart disease in clinical practice. Heart 1998; **80 suppl 2:** S1-S29.

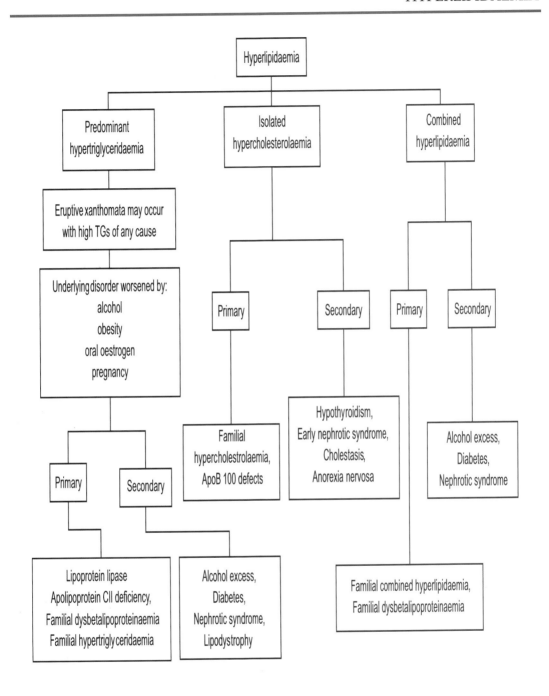

Hyperpigmentation of the skin

Hyperpigmentation in endocrine disorders

Generalised increased skin pigmentation is most intense on light exposed areas, in flexures, at sites of friction and pressure, in the creases of the palms and soles, and on all mucous membranes. The pattern is not specific and the possibility of Addison's disease should be considered in any case of increased pigmentation. In autoimmune Addison's disease, patches of non-pigmented skin (vitiligo) may also be present. The principal endocrine causes of hyperpigmentation are:

- adrenal failure
- acromegaly
- Cushing's syndrome
- hyperthyroidism
- phaeochromocytoma
- carcinoid syndrome
- high dose ACTH therapy.

Chloasma or melasma

This is a blotchy pigmentation of the cheeks and pigmentation of the nipples and linea alba. It is almost invariable in pregnancy and is particularly noticeable in dark haired women. It can also occur with oral contraceptive use and be associated with menstruation.

Hyperpigmentation in malignant disease

The principal types are:

- diffuse pigmentation in cachexia
- diffuse slaty-blue colour due to melanoma
- acanthosis nigricans (localised to the flexures). Acanthosis nigricans is characteristically associated with stomach cancer, but cases are frequently seen in subjects with insulin resistance e.g. polycystic ovary syndrome and acromegaly.

Hyperpigmentation in general medical disorders

Causes include:

- chronic infections and/or malnutrition (since they frequently co-exist) e.g. tuberculosis, Whipple's disease
- scleroderma
- chronic renal failure
- anaemia due to vitamin B12 deficiency (in contrast to vitiligo associated with

pernicious anaemia)
- cirrhosis of the liver
- haemochromatosis
- dermatomyositis.

Pigmentation associated with nutritional deficiencies

The principal causes are:

- deficiencies of any of vitamins A, C, niacin, folate or B12
- malabsorption syndromes
- 'Vagabond's disease' ? post-inflammatory pigmentation.

Pigmentation associated with drugs

Drugs most commonly involved include:

- anti malarials
- arsenic
- phenothiazines, especially chlorpromazine
- phenytoin (pigmentation resembles chloasma).

Hyperuricaemia

Uric acid is the major breakdown product of the purines adenosine and guanosine. It is largely excreted in the urine and increased plasma urate is therefore due either to increased production or decreased excretion.

Primary hyperuricaemias

Lesch-Nyhan syndrome
This is due to an inherited deficiency of hypoxanthine-guanine phosphoribosyl transferase (HGPRT) which is one of the salvage pathways for purines.

Glucose 6-phosphatase deficiency (von Gierke's, glycogen storage disease type I)
Hyperuricaemia is frequently present in this condition and is probably due to the co-existence of hyperlactataemia which inhibits uric acid excretion. Other biochemical features include hypoglycaemia and increased plasma concentrations of cholesterol, triglycerides, pyruvate and lactate. Gouty arthritis does not usually present until after the first decade.

Essential hyperuricaemia

Essential, or primary, hyperuricaemia is due to either overproduction (10-20%) or underexcretion (80-90%) of uric acid. Uric acid clearance of < 6 mL/min (normal 6 - 11) and daily excretion of < 3.6 mmol/24 hours is suggestive of renal under-excretion. In subjects with raised plasma urate, the daily urinary excretion may be normal.

NB: acute attacks of gout can be precipitated by treatment with allopurinol or probenecid.

Causes of secondary hyperuricaemia

Increased turnover of purines
- myeloproliferative disorders and chemotherapy resulting in massive cell breakdown e.g. lymphomas
- starvation
- psoriasis.

Reduced uric acid excretion
- renal failure
- thiazide diuretics (which inhibit renal excretion of uric acid)
- salicylates
- pyrazinamide, ethambutol
- chronic lead poisoning
- increased plasma ketones and lactate.

Uncertain mechanism
- hypothyroidism
- hyperparathyroidism
- eclampsia.

Pseudogout

This is clinically similar to gout but the crystals deposited are calcium pyrophosphate.

Renal stones

About 20% of subjects with clinical gout have urinary uric acid stones; 10% of renal stones are composed of urate.

Fallacies about gout

Gout is due to the precipitation of uric acid crystals within a joint and the plasma urate concentration is of no diagnostic use in the differential diagnosis of a monoarthropathy. Plasma urate concentration is useful in determining the therapeutic value of allopurinol and uricosuric agents.

The typical gout sufferer in 18th century caricatures had a high alcohol and protein diet. This is a misleading picture. However, in a predisposed individual, diet may increase the likelihood of an attack since high protein diets do create a purine load to be metabolised and ethanol may be metabolised to lactate which inhibits uric acid excretion into urine.

Metabolic acidosis

Metabolic acidosis is a common clinical problem and is often caused by diabetes, renal failure or poisoning. However, it can cause diagnostic difficulties, particularly in severe acute illness and where the aetiology is not obvious. It is vital that its diagnosis is considered in the clinical context with attention given to history (especially of drugs) and physical signs.

Metabolic acidosis is characterised by a raised $[H^+]$ and a low/normal arterial pCO_2 (in contrast with respiratory acidosis where the pCO_2 is high). A low derived bicarbonate or low plasma total CO_2 accompanies the raised $[H^+]$.

The raised $[H^+]$ stimulates the respiratory centre and hyperventilation occurs with a slight rise in pO_2. Hyperventilation reduces pCO_2 and hence some of the potential acid burden on the body and acts to compensate for the metabolic acidosis. Complete compensation does not occur (i.e. the $[H^+]$ remains elevated) and the extent of the compensation will be limited in patients with an underlying impairment of respiratory function.

Some confusion may occur in patients admitted with 'collapse' and *in extremis*. Cardiorespiratory collapse will result in a mixed acidosis due to a peripheral metabolic acidosis secondary to poor perfusion and a respiratory acidosis secondary to poor ventilation, resulting in a raised $[H^+]$ and raised $pCO2$

Anion gap = $[Na^+ + K^+] - [Cl^- + HCO_3^-]$ Usual reference range 12-20 mmol/L

Causes of lactic acidosis	
Type A – tissue hypoxia	severe hypoxia, severe anaemia, shock, haemorrhage, hypotension, congestive cardiac failure
Type B – no evident tissue hypoxia	diabetes, liver failure, seizures, leukaemia, tumours, thiamin deficiency, ethanol, methanol, ethylene glycol, salicylate, paracetamol glucose 6-phosphatase deficiency, fructose 1,6-diphosphatase deficiency

An elevated plasma lactate does not always indicate lactic acidosis. A raised plasma lactate may rise as a consequence of alkalosis since in alkalosis there is:

- increased glycolysis

- increased oxygen demand due to lactate induced vasodilatation

- impaired mitochondrial respiration.

These factors are exacerbated by increasing oxygen debt due to:

- reduced oxygen delivery due to the shift in the oxyhaemoglobin dissociation curve

- further anaerobic lactate accumulation

- hypoventilation (secondary to alkalosis).

Generalised muscle weakness

Weakness is a feature of a wide spectrum of disorders and this algorithm is only intended as a simplified approach as the diagnostic paths taken will be completely governed by the clinical history and physical signs. There are few specific diagnostic tests for this symptom and many disorders may non-specifically make a patient feel weak.

Metabolic causes of myopathy

Familial periodic paralysis

Diabetes

Hyper- and hypothyroidism

Hypercalcaemia

Hypocalcaemia

Hypomagnesaemia

Hypophosphataemia

Renal tubular acidosis

Cushing's syndrome

Rhabdomyolysis

McArdle's disease

Familial myoglobinuria

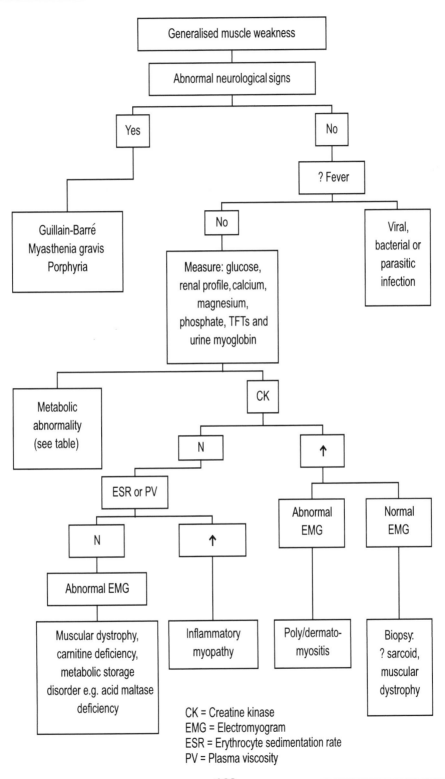

CK = Creatine kinase
EMG = Electromyogram
ESR = Erythrocyte sedimentation rate
PV = Plasma viscosity

Porphyria

The porphyrias are usually considered a difficult category of diseases as they are rare and because there appears to be no apparent relationship between the symptomatology and the biochemical pathways. Despite this, the diagnosis can only be made if there is a high index of suspicion with all cases of photosensitivity, abdominal pain or unexplained neurological disorders e.g. status epilepticus and encephalopathies.

The porphyrias can be classified into those disorders causing acute crises, photosensitivity or a combination. Photosensitivity may present either as acute painful swelling of the exposed skin or as fragility of exposed skin. This latter feature may appear as repeated tears on minimal trauma, easy bruising or multiple tiny scars.

If an acute porphyria is suspected, urine samples should be taken for urgent analysis of PBG, δ-ALA and total porphyrins. Porphyrins are stable in light-protected containers. Since an accurate diagnosis is essential and porphyrins are not frequently assayed in most routine laboratories, it is recommended that a specialist laboratory is approached.

Clinical presentation of the porphyrias

	Porphyrias causing acute abdominal or neurological crises	Porphyrias causing mixed symptomatology	Porphyrias causing photosensitivity
Disorder	Acute intermittent porphyria	Variegate porphyria	Congenital erythropoetic porphyria
		Hereditary coproporphyria	Porphyria cutanea tarda
			Erythropoetic protoporphyria
Symptoms	Acute crises characteristically cause abdominal pain but neuropsychiatric disturbances including status epilepticus, unexplained encephalopathy mood disturbances and peripheral neuropathies may be presenting features.	Acute and neuro-psychiatric symptoms are the usual presenting features. Photosensitivity (30%) may mimic PCT or may be present only during acute episodes.	Patients with EPP are likely to exhibit classical photosensitivity with painful swollen reddening of exposed skin, whereas PCT patients may only show pigmentation and/or scars in a light exposed distribution, i.e. on malar regions of the face and backs of the hands.

	Porphyrias causing acute abdominal or neurological crises	Porphyrias causing mixed symptomatology	Porphyrias causing photosensitivity
Investigations	Random urine sample for urgent analysis of PBG and δ-ALA to confirm the presence of an acute porphyria	During remission send urine and stool samples in light protected container. During acute episodes send random urine for PBG and δ-ALA.	Send urine and stool samples in light-protected container if EPP is suspected send heparin/EDTA blood sample (notify laboratory).

Investigations appropriate for symptoms

Symptoms	Diagnosis	Diagnostic test
Acute attack	Acute intermittent porphyria	PBG and δ-ALA markedly (i.e. > 10 fold) raised during an attack and are characteristically raised during remission. Most patients have reduced activity of erythrocyte PBG deaminase (but only a proportion of gene carriers develop clinical disease).
Acute attack	Variegate porphyria	Increased stool protoporphyrin and urine coproporphyrin. Characteristic plasma fluorescence @ 626 nm.
Acute attack	Hereditary coproporphyria	Increased stool coproporphyrin III and no increase in stool protoporphyrin. Increased urine coproporphyrin.
Fragility of exposed skin	Porphyria cutanea tarda	Increased urinary uroporphyrin and stool isocoproporphyrin.
Acute pain on exposure of skin to sunlight	Congenital erythropoetic porphyria	Massively increased uroporphyrin I.
	Erythropoetic protoporphyria	Increased erythrocyte zinc protoporphyrin. Reduced erythrocyte ferrochelatase activity.

Porphyria cutanea tarda

PCT is likely to be due to the coincidental association of several factors including liver toxins/disease and iron overload. A relationship with heterozygosity of the HFE haemochromatosis gene has been reported. In the past, the hepatic damage was usually caused by alcohol, however, nowadays in Western Europe, the majority of cases of PCT appear to be associated with hepatitis C and all patients should be tested for this.

Secondary porphyrias

Increased excretion of porphyrins in the urine and stools are seen in association with other disorders e.g. tyrosinaemia, lead poisoning, iron deficiency and alcoholism.

Symptoms similar to an acute attack may occur with lead poisoning and tyrosinaemia but in these cases the urine contains excess δ-ALA but no PBG.

Drugs associated with porphyria

The list of drugs safe to use or essential to avoid is continually being revised and up to date information can be obtained from the following porphyria internet sites:

http://www.uq.edu.au/porphyria

http://www.uct.ac.za/depts/liver/php.htm

Reference

Elder GH. Worwood M. Mutations in the hemochromatosis gene, porphyria cutanea tarda, and iron overload. Hepatology. 1998; **27:** 289-91.

Hormone replacement therapy

In all cases the most important guide to the adequacy of hormone replacement is the patient's symptomatic response. In some cases biochemical monitoring may help to guide dosing adjustment.

Thyroid hormone replacement

Thyroid hormone replacement therapy is almost always given in the form of thyroxine (T4). In health, 20% of tri-iodothyronine (T3) is produce by the thyroid gland rather than by conversion of T4 in the periphery, but in patients on T4 replacement all T3 is produced by peripheral conversion, and so circulating T4 concentations may need to be maintained slightly above the normal reference range to generate adequate tissue T3 concentrations.

In primary hypothyroidism, TSH is a useful guide to the adequacy of thyroxine replacement, the aim being to maintain it within the bottom half of the reference range i.e. 0.5-3.5 mU/L. However, some patients do not respond symptomatically until the TSH is suppressed and in this case thyroid hormone concentrations should be kept within the upper half of the reference ranges. It should be noted that otherwise healthy subjects who have a suppressed TSH have a high prevalence of atrial fibrillation and full suppression in patients on thyroxine therapy probably should be avoided.

In those with secondary hypothyroidism, measurement of TSH is of no value. Replacement should be based on symptoms, with an aim of keeping thyroid hormone concentrations within the upper half of the reference range.

Adrenal steroid replacement

There is no single test to ensure adequate cortisol replacement. If it is thought that the replacement dose is incorrect, a cortisol day curve can help to tailor doses to resemble a physiological profile.

In patients with primary adrenal insufficiency mineralocorticoid replacement should result in normal levels of plasma renin activity.

Gonadal steroid replacement

When oestrogen replacement therapy is used for relief of menopausal symptoms, response should be judged by the symptomatic response. FSH is useful for diagnosing the menopause but is not reduced by HRT.

Longer term oestrogen replacement therapy has been advocated for the prevention of osteoporosis in post-menopausal women on the basis of large cohort and case-control studies, despite a probable increased risk of breast cancer and venous thromboembolism. The case for using HRT to reduce the rate of ischaemic heart disease remains unproven. Recently the HERS study, a randomised, placebo controlled study of oestrogen replacement in post-menopausal women with ischaemic heart disease failed to show any beneficial effect in reducing cardiovascular events. Even in studies where benefit has apparently been demonstrated, the effects attenuate once oestrogen replacement is stopped, the risk of ischaemic heart disease and osteoporotic fracture increasing to control levels after 5-10 years.

When women use oestrogen replacement therapy for prevention of osteoporosis the response can be monitored using bone densitometry.

Testosterone replacement therapy in males should be assessed on the basis of symptomatic response. Ideally the dosage and frequency of intramuscular administration should be adjusted to ensure that plasma testosterone concentrations remain in the midnormal range one week after injection and within the normal range until the next dose. For patches, plasma testosterone should be measured 24-48 hours after patch application. Once physiological steady states have been achieved, patients should be reassessed every six months. Screening for lipids and prostate specific antigen (PSA) should probably be performed annually, PSA having been measured prior to commencing testosterone therapy.

Low-dose testosterone replacement (100 mg implant 4-6 monthly) may be indicated in post-menopausal women with diminished libido irrespective of whether they are receiving oestrogen replacement therapy.

Monitoring vitamin D therapy
Vitamin D derivatives are used for the treatment of chronic hypocalcaemia, in combination with 1.5 - 2 g of calcium supplements. Alfacalcidol (1α-hydroxycholecalciferol) and calcitriol (1,25-dihydroxycholecalciferol) are most commonly used. These agents have a short half-life (about six hours) and produce an optimal effect within three days.

Initially, plasma calcium concentrations should be checked twice weekly and the dose of vitamin D adjusted accordingly until a steady state is achieved. Thereafter, calcium concentrations should be checked frequently, at most three monthly, and renal function and urinary calcium excretion should be assessed 6-12 monthly. The aim should be to maintain plasma calcium concentrations towards the lower half of the reference range, and to ensure normal urinary calcium excretion. Patients should be warned of the symptoms of hypercalcaemia. If hypercalcaemia occurs, the drug should be stopped and intravenous rehydration commenced. Plasma calcium will rapidly normalize owing to the short half-life of these agents.

Monitoring should be performed more frequently during pregnancy, since the requirements for vitamin D therapy may double or triple towards the end of pregnancy. Post-partum the dose should be reduced to the pre-pregnancy level if not breast feeding, or to half the pre-pregnancy dose if breast feeding, increasing to the equivalent dose on cessation of breast feeding. This is because of the increase in endogenous vitamin D production during lactation.

References

Hulley S, Grady D, Bush T, Furberg C, Herrington D, Riggs B, Vittinghoff E. Randomized trial of estrogen plus progestin for secondary prevention of coronary heart disease in postmenopausal women. Heart and Estrogen/progestin Replacement Study (HERS) Research Group. JAMA 1998; **280:** 605-13.

Sawin CT, Geller A, Wolf PA, Belanger AJ, Baker E, Bacharach P, Wilson PWF, Benjamin EJ, D'Agostino RB. Low serum thyrotropin concentrations as a risk factor of atrial fibrillation in older persons. New Engl J Med 1994; **331:** 1249-52.

Bone pain

Bone pain may result from a pathological fracture, due either to metabolic bone disease or malignancy, or from certain metabolic bone diseases in the absence of overt fracture, such as osteomalacia, hyperparathyroidism or Paget's disease. Osteoporosis does not cause pain in the absence of fracture.

If the fracture has the characteristics of a fragility fracture, the bone scan shows a single focus, or other causes for fracture are excluded, osteoporosis should be considered and bone densitometry performed if uncertainty exists. Secondary causes of osteoporosis should be excluded if this has not already been done.

In the majority of cases, routine biochemical analyses and isotope bone scan should be performed as a first line investigation in all patients.

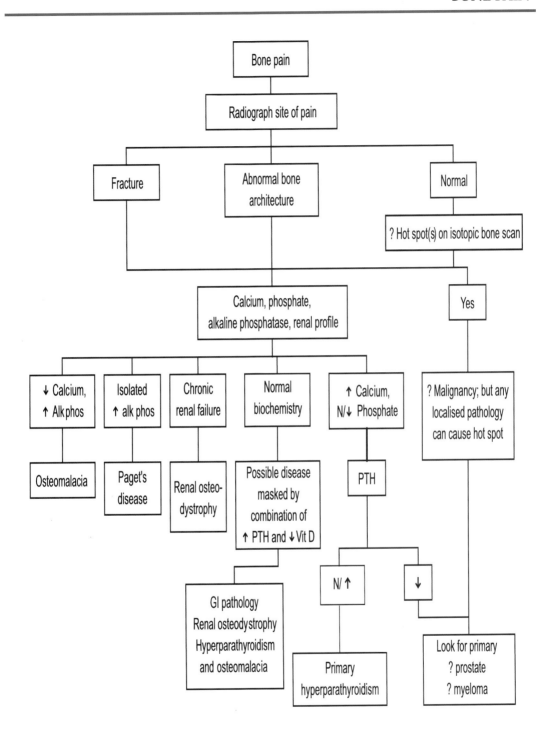

Osteomalacia and rickets

Diagnostic features

In osteomalacia there is a normal bony matrix which is undercalcified. Rickets is the clinical sign of deformation at the bony epiphyses if calcium deficiency occurs during bone growth. Osteomalacia is the clinical description of signs that occur after epiphyseal closure. The symptoms of both are: bone pain, fractures and proximal myopathy. 'Looser's zones' are seen on X-ray when there is loss of cortical bone.

Biochemical findings

In cases due to abnormalities of vitamin D, there is hypocalcaemia due to low vitamin D and secondary hyperparathyroidism. This is turn causes an increase in renal excretion of phosphate and reduced loss of calcium in the urine leading to hypophosphataemia. Plasma alkaline phosphatase activity is increased as a result of increased osteoblastic activity.

Causes of osteomalacia

• Malnutrition due to poor diet of calcium, phosphate and/or vitamin D.

• Malabsorption of calcium, phosphate and/or vitamin D due to gastrointestinal disease.

• Poor synthesis of vitamin D due to liver or renal failure i.e. failure of 1α-hydroxylation of vitamin D3 or, rarely, inadequate sunlight.

• Increased inactivation of vitamin D by anticonvulsants.

• Vitamin D resistance syndromes (rare).

• Renal tubular loss of phosphate due to X-linked hypophosphataemic rickets, tumour-induced phosphaturia and miscellaneous causes e.g. renal tubular acidosis and Fanconi syndrome.

Osteoporosis

Osteoporosis is due to a primary loss of bone matrix with no secondary osteoblastic repair process. Plasma concentrations of calcium and phosphate, and alkaline phosphatase activities are normal.

Risk factors for osteoporotic fracture
- Previous fragility fracture - suggests established, but possibly unrecognised, disease
- Liver disease
- Excessive alcohol ingestion
- Malabsorption
- Thyrotoxicosis
- Rheumatoid arthritis
- Male hypogonadism
- Primary hyperparathyroidism
- Myeloma
- Anorexia nervosa
- Prolonged immobilisation
- Current or planned long term oral corticosteroid use (> 7.5 mg prednisolone per day for three months or more), Cushing's syndrome
- Family history of osteoporosis (especially maternal hip fracture)
- Early surgical or natural menopause (before age 45 years)
- Pre-menopausal amenorrhoea > three months not due to pregnancy
- Hysterectomy, with at least one ovary conserved, before age 45 – this may affect ovarian function.

A diagnostic DEXA scan should be considered in:
Women with:
- oestrogen deficiency (menopause, hysterectomy before 45yrs, prolonged secondary amenorrhoea or primary hypogonadism), if HRT contraindicated and in those who are uncertain about or do not wish to take HRT

- clinical risk factors for osteoporosis (see above) at menopause to identify future fracture risk only in those who are uncertain about or do not wish to take HRT.

Men and women with:
- possible secondary osteoporosis (see risk factors above) all men, and women not taking or uncertain about HRT

- previous low impact fracture if there is uncertainty about diagnosis

- height loss or kyphosis if there is uncertainty about diagnosis i.e. no vertebral deformity on plain radiograph

- X-ray evidence of osteopenia if there is uncertainty about diagnosis

- corticosteroid use (> 7.5 mg daily for three months or more) to identify fast bone losers or to monitor therapy.

Patients on steroids

Controversy exists about the approach to corticosteroid-induced osteoporosis. The guidelines proposed by the National Osteoporosis Society suggest:

- for individuals more than 65 years who take > 15 mg prednisolone daily – treat for osteoporosis

- for others, consider risk factors and perform DEXA scan if present

- If one, or more, strong risk factors are present or bone mineral density $T < -1.5$ – treat for osteoporosis

- if no risk factors, repeat DEXA after 1 year and treat if bone loss > 4% at spine or > 7% at hip.

References

DoH website: http://www.open.gov.uk/doh/osteop.htm August 1998

Guidelines on the prevention and management of corticosteroid induced osteoporosis, National Osteoporosis Society, 1998

Nutrition

Clinical malnutrition can result from a number of factors including an inability to eat, poor diet, malabsorption and loss of nutrients. An imbalance between intake and expenditure results in a negative nitrogen balance, muscle wasting and widespread cellular dysfunction causing complications such as infection, poor wound healing, changes in drug metabolism, prolonged hospitalisation and increased mortality.

Nutritional deficiency is particularly likely to occur in patients unable to eat after surgery or cancer treatments and in those with gastrointestinal disorders. The overall incidence of malnutrition in hospitalised patients is of the order of 40-50%.

Assessment of basal metabolic rate (BMR) in healthy subjects

Estimates of BMR and energy expenditure are based on healthy ambulant subjects. Hospitalised patients will have considerably greater energy requirements, due for example to the effects of fever and inflammatory processes. These patients will need an adequate energy supply to minimise catabolic loss of muscle.

BMR in healthy subjects		
	age (years)	BMR (kcal/24h)
men	10-18	$17.5 \times W + 651$
	18-30	$15.3 \times W + 679$
	30-60	$11.6 \times W + 879$
	>60	$13.5 \times W + 487$
women	10-18	$12.2 \times W + 746$
	18-30	$14.7 \times W + 496$
	30-60	$8.7 \times W + 829$
	>60	$10.5 \times W + 596$
W = weight in kilograms		

Daily energy expenditure in healthy subjects		
	activity level	daily energy expenditure
men	inactive	BMR x 1.30
	light	BMR x 1.55
	moderate	BMR x 1.78
	heavy	BMR x 2.10
women	inactive	BMR x 1.30
	light	BMR x 1.56
	moderate	BMR x 1.64
	heavy	BMR x 1.82

Assessment of nutritional state

Advanced malnutrition is easy to recognise but it is difficult to define early malnutrition with the aim of evaluating the requirement for nutritional support. The most practical method is to use a bedside technique based on history taking and clinical examination which uses subjective criteria - the subjective global assessment.

Subjective global assessment of nutrition (SGA):

1. *Weight change:* overall loss over past 6 months in kg and % loss over past two weeks.

2. *Dietary intake change (duration in weeks):* gradation from no change to starvation.

3. *Gastrointestinal symptoms that have persisted for more than two weeks:* no symptoms, anorexia, nausea and vomiting.

4. *Functional capacity:* optimal, duration and dysfunction, type (working, ambulatory, bedridden).

5. *Disease and its relation to nutritional requirements:* primary diagnosis, metabolic demand.

6. *Examination:* loss of subcutaneous fat, muscle wasting, dependent, oedema, ascites.

The subjective use of the criteria above can be used to form a nutritional assessment of an individual as: well nourished, mildly or severely malnourished. Despite the lack of a rigid scoring system, the SGA has been shown to be reproducible, to correlate with multiple measures of body composition and moreover, to be predictive of adverse clinical events. It should not be forgotten that obese patients, too, can be malnourished. Significant loss of metabolically active lean body mass i.e. muscle, may occur and be disguised by excess adipose tissue.

It should be noted that objective measures of nutritional status may give false impressions due to the effect of disease on the measurements, the delayed clinical response to nutritional depletion and because there are wide confidence limits for nutritional measurements.

Metabolic aspects of parenteral feeding

There are numerous techniques for nutritional support, including specific (e.g. protein) or general (all nutrients) supplementation of diet and enteral feeding by nasogastric or nasojejunal tube, percutaneous gastrostomy etc. Patients whose nutrient requirement cannot be met fully by enteral feeding, will require parental feeding either supplementary or as the sole source of nutrients (total parenteral nutrition).

All patients requiring nutritional support require monitoring, involving clinical assessment, anthropometric measurements (e.g. weight, skinfold thickness) and laboratory investigations. The latter are particularly important in parenteral nutrition, as nutients and a large volume of fluid are infused directly into the blood. Monitoring is required:

• to assess the adequacy of nutritional provision
• to detect metabolic complications.

Clinical monitoring: daily weight, vital signs, fluid input and output measurements, regular assessment for sepsis and oral hygiene.

Laboratory monitoring: haemoglobin, white cell count, glucose, potassium and phosphate (daily initially and subsequently twice weekly), biochemical liver tests including albumin, calcium, magnesium and triglycerides. Trace elements - zinc, copper and selenium weekly. In practice, the frequency of tests is often determined by the patient's overall clinical state or underlying illness rather than the need to monitor nutritional support. Stable patients on long-term e.g. home parenteral nutrition require routine monitoring only at much greater intervals e.g. 4-6 weekly. Measurements or vitamin A and E may be required in some patients. CRP

- since there are physiological changes in many of the above biological markers with degrees of inflammation, CRP can be used to evaluate the degree of pathophysiological interference.

Effect of illness on plasma micronutrient concentrations		
Analyte	Minor inflammation i.e. CRP ~ 20 mg/L	Major inflammation i.e. CRP 100-200 mg/L
Iron	decreased by 40%	decreased by 60-90%
Zinc	decreased by 10%	decreased by 40-60%
Selenium	decreased by 10%	decreased by 40-60%
Copper	increased by 10-15%	increased by 30%
Vitamin A	decreased by 30-40%	decreased by 30%
Vitamin E	negligible	decreased by 20-30%
Vitamin B6	no data	decreased by 40-50%

Complications: hyper- and hypoglycaemia, electrolyte disturbances especially of potassium, magnesium and phosphate, due either to the quantity administered or redistribution consequent on insulin-mediated glucose uptake. Trace element and vitamin deficiencies may be avoided by regular administration but cannot be reliably assessed by plasma concentrations in the presence of infection. Hypertriglyceridaemia may be due to excess infusion, endogenous production, reduced utilisation or synthesis from carbohydrate infused in excess of needs. Mild cholestatic abnormalities in biochemical liver tests are frequently seen but usually settle spontaneously once parenteral nutrition is discontinued, but excessive energy may produce a fatty liver with persistent elevation of transaminases. The administration of amino acids may give rise to a mild metabolic acidosis which if necessary can be combated by the use of potassium acetate rather than chloride.

References

Baker JP, Detsky AS, Wesson DE, Wolman SL, Stewart S, Whitewell B et al. Nutritional assessment: a comparison of clinical judgement and objective measurements. New Engl J Med 1982: **306**: 969-72.

Department of Health. Dietary reference values for Food, Energy and Nutrients for the United Kingdom. London, HMSO. 1991.

Galloway P, McMillan DC, Sattar N. The inflammatory response: relevance to biochemical nutritional monitoring of trace elements and vitamins. Ann Clin Biochem 2000; **37**: 289-97.

Part 2. Investigation Protocols

Aldosterone sampling protocols - 1 - first line tests

Indication
Conventional practice suggests that the diagnosis of hyperaldosteronism should be considered in hypertensive patients with spontaneous or diuretic-induced hypokalaemia. However, data from clinics that routinely screen hypertensive patients indicates that a number of patients would be undiagnosed on this basis since approximately 50% of patients with aldosterone secreting adenomas are normokalaemic.

Contraindications
None.

Principle
Since the renin-aldosterone axis is primarily regulated by renal blood flow. Subjects under investigation should, therefore, not be taking any drugs that interfere with fluid balance or potassium. Neither doxazosin or prazosin interfere and those subjects requiring hypotensive therapy should ideally be transferred to one of these agents. Secondly, it is essential for subjects to be normally hydrated and have an adequate oral intake of sodium. Hypokalaemia must be avoided since it suppresses aldosterone secretion. It is important to note that increasing oral sodium intake may cause a considerable increase in urinary potassium excretion.

Side effects
None

Preparation
Give potassium replacement (Slow K tabs) sufficient to raise plasma potassium into the reference range (3.5-5.5 mmol/L). Replacement should be stopped on the day of the test.

Ideally, all interfering drugs should be stopped, but this may be impractical and a best pragmatic approach is often to stop ACE inhibitors and β-blockers for two weeks and to avoid calcium-channel blockers on the day of the test, although Valloton states that the aldosterone/renin ratio is robust and antihypertensive therapy does not need to be stopped when the ratio is used as a first line test.

The optimal approach is to use either bethanidine or prazosin as neither appears to affect the renin-aldosterone axis.

Drug	Physiological effect	Time for effect to be lost
ACE inhibitors	increase plasma renin activity (PRA), reduce aldosterone	2 weeks
β-blockers	reduce PRA more than aldosterone	2 weeks
Calcium channel blockers	reduce aldosterone, stimulate renin production	2 weeks
Diuretics	increase PRA and aldosterone	2 weeks
Hypokalaemia	inhibits aldosterone secretion	
NSAIDs	retain sodium, reduce PRA, ?effect on aldosterone	2 weeks
Oestradiol	increase renin substrate	6 weeks
Spironolactone	increase PRA, variable effect on aldosterone	2 weeks

Requirements
• Lithium heparin tube.

Blood samples should be taken rapidly to the laboratory but not on ice as PRA is measured by the activity of renin and at 4°C the inactive renin precursor is maximally converted to active renin.

Procedure
Samples should optimally be taken at 08:00 h when aldosterone is physiologically at its peak concentration.

The patient should remain seated for five minutes prior to venepuncture.

Random blood sample (10 mL lithium heparin tube) for PRA, aldosterone and potassium.

Interpretation
High aldosterone and suppressed plasma renin activity indicate primary hyperal-

dosteronism. Some patients with renal disease may give similar results.

Sensitivity and specificity

This test can only be a first line guide to the diagnosis of hyperaldosteronism. If the diagnosis is still unclear return to the hyperaldosteronism flow chart for second line dynamic tests.

References

Edwards CRW. Primary mineralocorticoid excess syndromes. In: DeGroot LJ et al. (eds.). Endocrinology. Philadelphia. Saunders: 3rd ed 1995; 1775-1803.

Gordon RD. Mineralocorticoid hypertension. Lancet 1994; **344:** 240-3.

McKenna TJ, Sequeira SJ, Heffernan A, Chambers J, Cunningham S. Diagnosis under random conditions of all disorders of the renin-aldosterone axis, including primary hyperaldosteronism. J Clin Endocrinol Met 1991; **73:** 952-7.

Valloton MB. Primary hyperaldosteronism. Part I Diagnosis of primary hyperaldosteronism. Clin Endocrinol (Oxf) 1996; **45:** 47-52.

Aldosterone sampling protocols - 2 - postural studies

Indication
Postural studies used to be the mainstay for the differential diagnosis between aldosterone-producing adenomas and adrenal hyperplasia; in the latter there is a rise in aldosterone on standing whereas with tumours there is a fall. However, it is now recognised that about one-third of aldosterone-producing adenomas are angiotensin- sensitive and respond to upright posture by a rise in the concentration of aldosterone, whereas the other half will not. In view of this, few authorities now recommend their use.

Preparation
Ideally, all interfering drugs should be stopped, but this is impractical and a best pragmatic approach is often to stop ACE inhibitors and β-blockers for two weeks before the test. The optimal approach is to use either bethanidine or prazosin, neither of which appear to affect the renin-aldosterone axis.

Requirements
• Three Lithium heparin tubes.

Blood samples should be taken rapidly to the laboratory but not on ice as plasma renin activity (PRA) is measured by the activity of renin and at 4°C the inactive renin precursor is maximally converted to active renin.

Procedure
Subjects should be placed on a diet containing at least 100-150 mmol/24h sodium and 75-125 mmol/24h potassium. This should be assessed by at least one 24h urine collection prior to the investigation. It is essential that the subject should not rise from bed after 22:00 h the night prior to investigation for any reason to ensure that basal levels of analytes are measured in the first sample.

08:30 h before breakfast	take 10mL blood into a lithium heparin tube for cortisol, PRA and aldosterone. The patient should not return to bed (they may sit, stand or walk) until the midday sample is taken.
09:00 h before breakfast	take 10 mL blood into a lithium heparin tube for cortisol, PRA and aldosterone.
12:00 h before midday meal	take 10 mL blood into a lithium heparin tube for cortisol, PRA and aldosterone.

Interpretation

The baseline sample is taken to confirm the presence of hyperaldosteronism and to evaluate the aldosterone:PRA ratio under the controlled conditions on which the reference data has been collected.

The second sample is taken to establish that the effect of posture is to cause a physiological rise in PRA. No change in PRA suggests that aldosterone secretion is autonomous.

The midday sample may help classify the nature of the adenoma. Aldosterone producing adenomas are either angiotensin-dependent or ACTH-dependent. The former is suggested by a midday concentration of aldosterone which rises to twice the 08:30 h value whereas a fall of 50% suggests ACTH dependence. The latter requires confirmation by assessment of the physiological fall in ACTH at midday by demonstration of a fall in plasma cortisol from 08:30 h to 12:00 noon.

The aldosterone secretion in bilateral adrenal hyperplasia is generally angiotensin-dependent and will rise in the midday sample.

Aldosterone-producing adenoma are typically described as showing a fall in aldosterone between the recumbent and ambulant samples. This is consistent with an ACTH-dependent, or angiotensin-unresponsive, adenoma.

Patients with familial aldosteronism type 1 (glucocorticoid-suppressible) also show a fall in aldosterone in the midday sample.

References

Feltynowski T, Ignatowska-Switalska H, Wocial B, Lewandowski J, Chodakowska J, Jaruszewic W. Postural stimulation test in patients with aldosterone producing adenomas. Clin Endocrinol (Oxf) 1994; **41:** 309-14.

Gordon RD, Hamlet SM, Tunny TJ, Klemm SA. Aldosterone-producing adenomas responsive to angiotensin pose problems with diagnosis. Clin Exp Pharmacol Physiol 1987; **14:** 175-9.

Gordon RD. Mineralocorticoid hypertension. Lancet 1994; **344:** 240-3.

Short F, James VHT. Primary hyperaldosteronism in England and Wales: a review of the use of a supraregional assay service laboratory for the measurement of aldosterone and plasma renin activity. Ann Clin Biochem 1991; **28:** 218-25.

Ammonium chloride acidification test for renal tubular acidosis

> This test is potentially dangerous and must be undertaken with great care.
> It should NOT be performed if the urine is alkaline in the presence of a metabolic acidosis, in patients with liver disease or in patients taking alkali replacement.
>
> Bacterial urine infection may give a falsely high pH due to urea hydrolysis.
>
> This test should not be performed in hypokalaemia or hypercalcaemia as these conditions interfere with tubular function and may mimic RTA.

Indication
Renal tubular acidosis is characterised by an hyperchloraemic acidosis with a normal anion gap. The diagnosis is already established if urine is not maximally acidified (pH > 5.5) despite a metabolic acidosis (plasma bicarbonate < 17.5 mmol/L) in the presence of normal renal function.

Principle
Ammonium chloride is converted in the liver to urea with the consumption of bicarbonate. The bicarbonate is replaced by renal synthesis with excretion of hydrogen ions. This test stresses the ability of the kidneys to excrete acid and any failure will result in a metabolic acidosis.

Side effects
Most patients who take ammonium chloride will feel a degree of nausea, abdominal discomfort and mild diarrhoea. Some patients will vomit but this can be reduced by allowing a longer ingestion period of two hours.

Preparation
No specific preparation is required though the patient must fast on the morning prior to the test.

Requirements
- Ammonium chloride (0.1 g/kg body weight).
- Six urine collecting vessels.
- Two lithium heparin blood tubes.

Procedure
General management
If possible keep the patient upright or ambulant during test. Food and drink may be given as required. From the moment the test is started, all urine must be collected for

at least the next 8 hours. Each specimen must be placed in a separate container and clearly labelled with the patient's name and the time of collection. Each specimen should be sent to the laboratory immediately.

	The patient should be fasting and should be weighed prior to the onset of the test. The first urine passed should be collected for measurement of pH. Out-patients may need to be given 300-400mL water to obtain this specimen. pH < 5.5 excludes almost all subjects with type 1 RTA. This result should be obtained prior to starting the test.
09:00 h	Collect a mid stream urine specimen and an anaerobic heparinised free-flowing venous blood sample (as for arterial blood gas determination) and send to the laboratory on ice for estimation of pH and bicarbonate. It is important that forearm exercise and venous occlusion are avoided since both result in a raised pH.
09:05 h	The patient should eat breakfast with ammonium chloride (0.1g/kg body weight). This may be given disguised with syrup or jam or in solution with iced water. The total dose should be taken over a period of two hours to reduce the degree of gastric irritation. If the total dose cannot be consume,d note the exact quantity on the request card. It will be necessary to repeat the test if the patient vomits all/the majority of the ammonium chloride.
13:15 h	Take a second venous blood sample and send to the laboratory on ice.
09:15 h to 17:00 h	Collect all urine passed. Samples should be collected at hourly intervals and periods of longer than two hours should be avoided - this should be achieved by ensuring that approximately 200 mL are drunk hourly. Any spillages should be accurately recorded.

Interpretation

Normal subjects should produce at least one urine specimen with a pH < 5.3 and have a rate of ammonia excretion in the region of 1 mmol/min/kg. The plasma TCO_2 should fall by approximately 4 mmol/L and the pH by 0.05 units.

In neonates, it is normal for the urine pH to be 6-7 for the first week of life and a more adult pattern develops afterwards. During the first year of life the renal threshold for bicarbonate is relatively low at approximately 17-19 mmol/L whereas in adults it is 20-26 mmol/L.

• *The urinary pH does not fall below 5.3 during the test.*
RTA type 1 is due to a distal tubular inability to excrete hydrogen ions against a gradient. This results in loss of potassium and hypokalaemia. Chronic acidosis results in calcium wasting and consequently renal stones. This form of RTA may be secondary to other disorders e.g. nephrocalcinosis and galactosaemia.

• *The urinary pH does fall below 5.3 during the test.*
RTA type 2 is often part of a generalised proximal tubular dysfunction (i.e. Fanconi syndrome) and is due to a partial failure to reabsorb bicarbonate (fractional clearance may be > 15%). Bicarbonate concentration falls to the level at which the tubules are able to absorb it completely (approximately 16-20 mmol/L). Hypokalaemia is a feature. Hypercalciuria occurs but renal stones are unusual. The urine is often not alkaline in the steady state (because of complete absorption of the reduced filtered load due to low plasma bicarbonate).

Diagnostic features include low plasma bicarbonate, alkaline urine, ability to acidify urine and requirement for high doses of bicarbonate to correct acidosis. It may be necessary to infuse bicarbonate to measure the threshold.

RTA type 4 is probably a distal tubular disorder. It is characterised by an acid urine during a metabolic acidosis. There is little bicarbonate wasting but poor urinary ammonia production and a high plasma potassium. Renal calcium stones do not develop and there is no Fanconi syndrome. It is often secondary to diabetic or hypertensive nephropathy. There is hyporeninaemic hypoaldosteronism even during extracellular volume depletion.

References

Caldas A, Broyer M, Dechaux M, Kleinknecht C. Primary distal tubular acidosis in childhood: clinical study and longterm follow-up of 28 patients. J Pediatr 1992; **121:** 233-41.

Oleesky D, Penny MD. Renal tubular acidosis. Ann Clin Biochem 1999; **36:** 408-22.

Tannen RL. The response of normal subjects to the short ammonium chloride test. Clin Sci 1971; **41:** 583-95.

Tannen RL, Falls WF Jr, Brackett NC Jr. Incomplete renal tubular acidosis: some clinical and physiological features. Nephron 1975; **15:** 111-23

Wrong O, Davies HEF. The excretion of acid in renal disease. Quart J Med 1959; **28:** 259-313

Calcium absorption test for hypercalciuria

Indication
This test is designed to differentiate between renal, absorptive or idiopathic hypercalciuria in subjects with renal calculi. It should be considered in males with urine calcium > 7.5 mmol/24h and females with urine calcium > 6.2 mmol/24h.

Contraindications
None.

Principle
Patients with post-absorptive hypercalciuria (AHC) by definition have normal fasting calciuria (defined as molar calcium:creatinine ratio < 0.23). Patients with AHC have excessive calciuria after an oral calcium load. Patients with type I AHC cannot lower their calciuria by dietary calcium restriction unlike those with type II AHC.

Side effects
None.

Preparation
No preparation required although patient should drink only water after 22:00 h on the night before the test.

Requirements
- Breakfast and calcium supplements to provide 1g calcium.
- Three 24h urine containers.
- One plain tube for blood collection.

Procedure
Patient is allowed free water overnight after 22:00 h.

0 h	• patient passes urine (sample 1: analysed for pH and microscopy)
	• blood sample taken without tourniquet for plasma urea, electrolytes, bicarbonate, calcium, phosphate, urate and PTH
0-2 h	• water is freely allowed (at least 0.5L) and all urine collected (sample 2: analysed for calcium, phosphate and creatinine)
2-6 h	• patient given breakfast with calcium supplement
	• water is freely allowed (at least 1L) and all urine collected for 4 h (sample 3: analysed for calcium, phosphate and creatinine)

Interpretation

	Absorptive hypercalciuria type I	Absorptive hypercalciuria type II	Absorptive hypercalciuria type III	Renal hypercalciuria
plasma calcium	N	N	N	N
plasma phosphate	N	N	-	N
plasma PTH	N	N	N	N
fasting calcium/ creatinine ratio (normal < 0.23 mmol/mmol)	< 0.23	< 0.23	> 0.36	> 0.36
urine calcium/ creatinine ratio following 1g load (normal < 0.46 mmol/mmol)	> 0.56	> 0.56	> 0.56	> 0.73
24h urine calcium on 400mg/24h diet (normal < 5 mmol)	> 5 mmol	< 5 mmol	> 5 mmol	> 5 mmol
Pathophysiology	hyper-absorption of calcium	diet-responsive hyper-calciuria	phosphate leak leads to decreased resorption of calcium	decreased renal resorption of calcium is primary defect

References

Coe FL, Parks JH, Asplin JR. The pathogenesis and treatment of kidney stones. New Eng J Med 1992; **327:** 1141-52.

Pak CYC, Kaplan R, Bone H, Townsend J, Waters O. A simple test for the diagnosis of absorptive, resorptive and renal hypercalciurias. New Eng J Med 1975; **292:** 497-500.

Wilkinson H. Clinical investigation and management of patients with renal stones. Ann Clin Biochem 2001; **38:** 180-7.

Clonidine test For phaeochromocytoma

Indication
The diagnosis of phaechromocytoma should initially be based on measurement of catecholamine excretion in two 24h urine collections. The clonidine test is required if there is strong clinical suspicion with non-diagnostic elevations of catecholamine excretion.

Contraindications
Medical anti-hypertensive therapy is not contra-indicated for this test but since there is a tendency for such treatment to lower the urinary excretion of (nor-)adrenaline, it is ideal to stop treatment for 24h prior to and during the test. The laboratory should be contacted to ascertain which, if any, drugs may interfere with the analytical detection of catecholamines.

Principle
Physiological catecholamine secretion is suppressed by clonidine whereas autonomous secretion by a tumour is not suppressed.

Side effects
Since clonidine may produce a profound fall in blood pressure, the subject should remain lying in bed throughout the night (21:00 - 07:00 h) except to pass urine.

Preparation
Patients should be admitted to hospital and should refrain from smoking or consuming caffeine (e.g. tea, coffee and cola drinks).

Requirements
- 0.3 mg clonidine.
- Two 24 h urine containers with acid preservative.

Procedure
Day 1: 21:00 h patient should empty his/her bladder and start an overnight collection of urine from 21:00 to 07:00 h using collection bottles with acid preservative.

Day 2: 21:00 h patient should empty his/her bladder.

Immediately afterwards 0.3mg clonidine should be taken orally.

An overnight collection of urine should be made from 21:00 - 07:00 h, using collection bottles with acid preservative.

Interpretation
In subjects both with and without hypertension, the effect of sleep and clonidine should lower urinary noradrenaline to < 58 nmol/mmol creatinine and urinary adrenaline to < 18 nmol/mmol creatinine.

Phaeochromocytoma should be considered in patients with higher values.

Reference
Macdougall IC, Isles CG, Stewart H, Ingles GC, Finlayson J, Thomson I, Lees KR, McMillan NC, Morley P, Ball SG. Overnight clonidine suppression test in the diagnosis and exclusion of pheochromocytoma. Am J Med 1988; **84:** 993-1000.

Low dose (1 mg) overnight dexamethasone suppression test

Indication
This should be the first line screening test for all subjects suspected of having Cushing's syndrome.

Contraindications
Patients on enzyme inducing drugs e.g. anticonvulsants and rifampicin, may rapidly metabolise dexamethasone and give a false positive result i.e. no suppression. Women on oestrogen therapy may fail to suppress adequately due to increased cortisol binding globulin. In these instances a higher dose of dexamethasone should be used.

Principle of test
In normal subjects, dexamethasone suppresses ACTH and therefore cortisol secretion. In Cushing's syndrome, there is incomplete suppression.

Side effects
None.

Preparation
This is an outpatient test and no patient preparation is necessary.

Requirements
- 1 mg dexamethasone tablet (the dose of dexamethasone for children is 15 μg/kg body weight).
- One plain blood tube.

Procedure
The patient takes 1 mg dexamethasone orally at 23:00 h and the following morning at exactly 09:00 h a blood sample (3 mL blood) is taken for plasma cortisol.

If the patient is collecting a 24 h urine sample for urinary free cortisol this should be completed before taking the dexamethasone.

Interpretation
A normal response is suppression of 09:00 h cortisol to < 50 nmol/L.

Sensitivity and specificity
Plasma cortisol normally falls after 09:00 h and false positive tests may occur if blood sampling is delayed.

Suppression in patients with Cushing's syndrome is rare with this test (2%). In the reported cases the patients have been shown to metabolise dexamethasone slowly and so achieve higher circulating concentrations than expected. If suppression occurs in a patient in whom there is strong clinical or biochemical evidence for Cushing's syndrome, this test should be repeated or a formal low dose (2 mg) dexamethasone test is performed.

Normal subjects rarely (2%) fail to suppress with overnight dexamethasone. False positives may occur with depression (30-50%) due to the development of a reversible glucocorticoid resistance, and in patients with severe systemic illness (10-20%). Patients with renal failure on dialysis may have false positive tests due to increased clearance of dexamethasone. The effect of chronic alcohol abuse is questioned by some but there are clearly described cases. Patients with simple obesity do not have an increased rate of false positive results.

The formal low dose (2 day) dexamethasone suppression test is slightly more specific. This test should probably be performed in a specialised endocrine unit.

References
Crapo L. Cushing's Syndrome: a review of diagnostic tests. Metabolism 1979; **28:** 955-79.

Wood P, Barth JH, Freedman DB, Perry L, Sheridan B. Evidence for the low dose dexamethasone suppression test to screen for Cushing's syndrome - recommendations for a protocol for UK biochemistry laboratories. Ann Clin Biochem 1997; **34:** 222-9.

Fasting test for the diagnosis of Gilbert's syndrome

Indication
Gilbert's syndrome is a relatively common cause of an unconjugated hyperbilirubi-naemia, often only becoming apparent when a minor elevation in plasma bilirubin detected during a mild illness does not fall with recovery. It is probably the result of a heterogeneous group of disorders some of which have a defect in the uptake of organic anion by the liver. Total bilirubin concentrations in this condition are usually in the range 20-50 µmol/L and rarely rise above 85 µmol/L. The total bilirubin fluc-tuates with intercurrent illness, physical exertion and stress.

The diagnosis of Gilbert's syndrome is predominantly by the exclusion of other conditions. This test may aid the diagnosis but does not give a definitive separation from hepatitis.

Contraindications
None.

Side effects
None.

Preparation
No specific patient preparation required.

Requirements
- Two biscuits.
- Two lithium heparin tubes.

Principle
Plasma bilirubin concentrations rise after fasting and other forms of metabolic stress e.g. surgery, fever or infection in all individuals, but the change is more marked in subjects with Gilbert's syndrome. The mechanism for this effect is unknown but is probably related to reduced hepatic clearance, rather than increased production, of bilirubin. This has been proposed to be due to competition by free fatty acids for the intracellular bilirubin binding protein.

Procedure
Day 1: take blood for total and unconjugated plasma bilirubin estimations:
    begin calorie restriction to 300 kcal per day (approximately 2 biscuits) .

Day 2: take blood for total and unconjugated plasma bilirubin estimations

Interpretation
Total bilirubin concentrations rise in normal individuals by approximately 60% after 48 h fasting, whereas in subjects with Gilbert's syndrome the total bilirubin concentration rises by approximately 90% after 24 h. The unconjugated bilirubin concentration rises by more than 110% after 24 h.

Reference
Owens D, Sherlock S. Diagnosis of Gilbert's syndrome: role of reduced caloric intake test. Br Med J 1973; **3:** 559

Fludrocortisone suppression test for hyperaldosteronism

Indication
This test is considered by some to be the definitive diagnostic procedure for hyper-aldosteronism.

Contraindications
The risk of sodium loading prohibits the use of this test in elderly subjects and those with severe hypertension.

Principle
Patients with hyperaldosteronism are in a state of salt retention. Therefore, further sodium loading with a sodium-retaining steroid will have no effect on plasma aldos-terone concentration. Adequate potassium needs to be administered to ensure that aldosterone secretion is not inhibited by hypokalaemia.

Side effects
See contraindications.

Preparation
Patient needs to be hospitalised for at least four days.

Requirements
- Fludrocortisone 0.1 mg tabs x 16.
- Slow Na (10 mmol) tabs x 36.
- Slow K (8 mmol) tabs - may need up to 200.
- Two Lithium heparin blood tubes.

Procedure
Day 1: plasma aldosterone should be measured midmorning. The subject should be sitting or standing for at least 30 min prior to venepuncture.

Fludrocortisone 0.1 mg is administered six hourly for four days.
Slow Na 3x10 mmol tabs are administered eight hourly for four days.
Slow K tabs administered in sufficient quantity to maintain a normal plasma potas-sium concentration.

Day 4: plasma aldosterone should be measured mid morning. The subject should be sitting or standing for at least 30 min prior to venepuncture.

Interpretation

Suppression of aldosterone excludes the diagnosis of primary hyperaldosteronism.

Sensitivity and specificity

Interpretation may be complicated by two factors if the patient remains recumbent that may result in a misleading lowering of aldosterone. First, aldosterone exhibits a diurnal rhythmn that is similar to, though less marked, than cortisol, with a fall in concentration as the day progresses. This is overcome by the effect of angiotensin if the patient is ambulant. Second, some tumours are responsive to angiotensin, and aldosterone will consequently be lowered by prolonged (e.g. > 2 hours) recumbency.

References

Gordon RD, Stowasser M, Klemm SA, Tunny TJ. Primary aldosteronism and other forms of mineralocorticoid hypertension. In: Swales JD (ed) Textbook of Hypertension. Oxford, Blackwells Science. 1994: 865-92.

Kem DC, Weinberger M, Gomez-Sanchez C, Kramer NJ, Lerman R, Furuyama S. et al. Circadian rhythm of plasma aldosterone concentration in patients with primary aldosteronism. J Clin Invest 1973; **52:** 2272-7.

Streeten DH, Tomycz N, Anderson GH. Reliability of screening methods for the diagnosis of primary hyperaldosteronism. Am J Med 1979; **67:** 403-13.

Frusemide test for hyperaldosteronism

Indication
This test can be used as a screening test for hyperaldosteronism in hypertensive patients since hypokalaemia is not a consistent finding.

Contraindications
The only risks are the potential effects of cessation of anti-hypertensive therapy.

Principle
Aldosterone is normally regulated by the renin-angiotensin system, which is in turn regulated by renal blood flow. If subjects are rendered hypovolaemic or hypotensive, the renin-angiotensin system should be stimulated. This does not occur in states of hyperaldosteronism.

Side effects
None.

Preparation
Ideally patients should stop taking diuretics, NSAIDs and certain anti-hypertensive agents (ACE inhibitors, β-blockers and calcium channel blockers) two weeks prior to this investigation, and oestradiol and spironolactone for six weeks. There are variable opinions on the absolute need for cessation of drug therapy, but results can be misleading in patients on spironolactone if this is not stopped adequately early, causing elevations in PRA even in patients with proven aldosterone-producing adenomata.

Requirements
- Two frusemide 40 mg tabs.
- Lithium heparin blood tube.

Procedure

Day 1 18:00 h	Give frusemide 40 mg orally
Day 2 09:00 h	Give frusemide 40 mg orally
09:00 - 11:00 h	Patient should remain upright and ambulant
11:00 h	Take blood for plasma renin activity

Interpretation

Failure of PRA to rise above 1.5 nmol/L/hr indicates primary hyperaldosteronism.

Sensitivity and specificity

This test separates all forms of mineralocorticoid excess from other causes of hypertension but does not indicate the cause i.e. bilateral adrenal hyperplasia, adrenal adenoma, idiopathic hyperaldosteronism, apparent mineralocorticoid excess, deoxycorticosterone-producing adenoma, etc.

References

Valloton MB. Primary aldosteronism. Part I Diagnosis of primary hyperaldosteronism. Clin Endocrinol (Oxf) 1996; **45:** 47-52.

Weinberger MH, Grim CE, Hollified JW, Kem DC, Ganguly A, Kramer NJ et al. Primary aldosteronism. Diagnosis, localization and treatment. Ann Intern Med 1979; **90:** 386-95.

Frusemide test for renal acidification defects

Indication

Renal tubular acidosis is characterised by an hyperchloraemic acidosis with a normal anion gap. The diagnosis is already established if urine is not maximally acidified (pH > 5.5) despite a metabolic acidosis (plasma bicarbonate < 17.5 mmol/L) in the presence of a normal renal function.

The main indication for this test of subtle renal tubular acidosis is in the differential diagnosis of the aetiology of renal stones when early morning urine has a pH > 5.5. It is a useful first line screening test for these patients.

Principle

Administration of frusemide results in an increase in the delivery of sodium ions to the distal renal tubules with a normal quantity of bicarbonate ions. In normal individuals A proportion of the extra sodium is reabsorbed in exchange for hydrogen ions resulting in an acid urine. This test stresses the distal tubules acidification capacity.

Side effects

None apart from a rapid diuresis – it is prudent to mention this to the patient.

Preparation

Patient is fasted overnight.
Spironolactone should be discontinued for 6 weeks prior to this test.

Requirements

- Nine urine sample containers.
- 40 mg frusemide tablet.

Procedure

Baseline urine sample for pH.

09:00 h oral administration of 40 mg frusemide.

09:30 - 13:00 h urine samples collected every 30 min (8 samples) and analysed for pH.

Interpretation

A normal response is a lowering of urine pH to less than 5.5 by 4 hours. A nadir in urinary pH should be achieved by 3-4 hours. The frequent urine pH measurements are necessary to avoid possible misclassification of some patients.

Sensitivity and specificity

The diagnostic performance of this test for the diagnosis of RTA in renal stone formers is: sensitivity 10%, specificity 82%, predictive value of a positive test 40%, predictive value of a negative test 100%. In view of the relatively poor predictive value of a positive test, patients with a positive test should progress to the ammonium chloride acidification test for confirmation.

Reference

Reynolds TM, Burgess N, Matanhelia S, Brain A, Penney MD. The frusemide test: simple screening test for renal acidification defect in urolithiasis. Br J Urol 1993; **72:** 153-6.

Glucagon test of the hypothalamo-pituitary axis

Indication
Assessment of pituitary-adrenal axis (GH and ACTH/cortisol). It is particularly useful when induction of hypoglycaemia using insulin is contraindicated.

Contraindications
The test should not be performed in subjects with hypothyroidism or severe adrenal failure i.e. 09:00 h cortisol < 100 nmol/L. The test is unreliable in patients with diabetes mellitus.

Hypoglycaemia may occur in: phaeochromocytoma, insulinoma, after prolonged starvation (> 48 hours) or glycogen storage diseases (because of inability to mobilise glycogen).

Principle of test
Glucagon stimulates the release of GH and ACTH by a hypothalamic mechanism and therefore indirectly stimulates cortisol secretion. Simultaneous administration of TRH and LHRH does not interfere with the effects of glucagon.

Intramuscular administration is essential as absorption via the subcutaneous route is unreliable.

Side effects
Some subjects feel unwell generally and about a third develop nausea and vomiting.

Preparation
The patient should be fasting from midnight but may drink water. The patient does not need to be continuously observed as hypoglycaemia is not provoked.

Requirements
• Glucagon: dose 1mg for adults (1.5 mg if > 90kg).

• Glucagon: dose for children is 15 µg/kg (maximum 1 mg).

• Indwelling cannula gauge 19.

• Three plain tubes.

Procedure

0 min	Take 3 mL blood into plain tube for cortisol and GH Immediately give glucagon intra-muscularly
150 min	Take 3 mL blood into plain tube for cortisol and GH
180 min	Take 3 mL blood into plain tube for cortisol and GH

Interpretation

An adequate cortisol response is defined as a rise of greater than 170 nmol/L to above 550 nmol/L. An adequate GH response is a rise to a value greater than 20 mU/L.

There is probably a blunted response in hypothyroidism and obesity.

Sensitivity and specificity

This test is generally considered to be a slightly less reliable test of the ability of the pituitary to secrete GH and ACTH than the insulin hypoglycaemia test, but its diagnostic efficacy is defined by the response to the IHT. It is an excellent alternative in patients who cannot tolerate hypoglycaemia because of epilepsy, ischaemic heart disease or hypopituitarism.

References

Mitchell ML, Byrne MJ, Sanchez Y, Sawin CT. Detection of growth-hormone deficiency: the glucagon stimulation test. N Eng J Med 1970; **282:** 539-41.

Orme SM, Peacey SR, Barth JH, Belchetz PE. Comparison of tests of stress-released cortisol secretion in pituitary disease. Clin Endocrinol (Oxf) 1996; **45:** 135-40.

Rao RAH, Spathis GS. Intramuscular glucagon as a provocative stimulus for the assessment of pituitary function: growth hormone and cortisol responses. Metabolism 1987; **36:** 658-63.

Glucagon test for glycogen storage disorders

Indication
This test is useful in the differential diagnosis of hypoglycaemia associated with ketosis.

Contraindications
This test should not be performed if there is hypoglycaemia or lactic acidosis at the time of the test.

Principle
Glucagon produces a rise in plasma glucose concentration by enhancing hepatic glycogenolysis. Normal subjects exhibit a rise in glucose but not in lactate unless there is a defect in gluconeogenesis.

Side effects
Some subjects feel unwell and a proportion develop nausea and vomiting. Sweating, palpitation, and rarely, loss of consciousness and convulsions may occur owing to severe hypoglycaemia.

Preparation
Prior to the test, measurement of glucose, urea and electrolytes for an assessment of anion gap should be carried out.

Requirements
- Five fluoride oxalate tubes for glucose and lactate.

- Glucagon for i.m. injection. Dose: 1 mg (adults), 15 µg/kg body weight (children)

See protocol for emergency treatment of hypoglycaemia during IHT/glucagon test

Procedure

Site an indwelling cannula in the antecubital fossa with good access for administration of glucose, if required

0 min	Take 2 mL blood for glucose and lactate Immediately afterwards administer glucagon as above.
30 min	Take 2 mL blood for glucose and lactate
60 min	Take 2 mL blood for glucose and lactate
90 min	Take 2 mL blood for glucose and lactate
120 min	Take 2 mL blood for glucose and lactate

Interpretation

Adults: in normal subjects there is a rise in plasma glucose of > 4 mmol/L. The greater rise seen in adults can be explained by the lesser disease severity.

Children: in normal subjects there is a rise in plasma glucose of > 2 mmol/L and a fasting or stimulated plasma lactate < 2.4 mmol/L.

GSD type	Glucose	Lactate	Effect of performing test post-prandially
Ia	Increased or decreased	Normal or increased	
Ib	Decreased	Increased	Greater fall in glucose
III	Normal	Normal	Glycaemic response
VI	Increased	Normal	Greater response

References

Pears JS, Jung RT, Hopwood D, Waddell ID, Burchell A. Glycogen storage disease diagnosed in adults. Quart J Med 1992; **82:** 207-22.

Dunger DB, Leonard JV. Value of the glucagon test in screening for hepatic glycogen storage disease. Arch Dis Child 1982; **57:** 384-9.

Oral glucose tolerance test for the diagnosis of diabetes mellitus

Indication
The diagnosis of diabetes is made on the basis of an elevated fasting or post-prandial plasma glucose concentration in a symptomatic subject, or two elevated concentrations in an asymptomatic subject. The oral glucose tolerance test is only used when such measurements are equivocal and is not required for diagnosis in the majority of patients.

Contraindication
This test should not be performed in patients with periodic hypokalaemic paralysis.

Principle
In normal individuals, pancreatic insulin secretion maintains blood glucose within a tight concentration range following an oral glucose load. Failure of insulin secretion, or resistance to the action of insulin, will result in an elevation in blood glucose.

Side effects
Some subjects feel nauseated and may have vaso-vagal symptoms during the test.

Preparation
Patients should fast for 10-16 h prior to this test but may drink small volumes of water. Subject's should eat their normal diet for 72 h before the test.

Requirements
• Adults: 75g anhydrous glucose in cold water. The solution should be chilled to improve palatability.

Lucozade ® is preferable to pure glucose solutions as it is less likely to make patients nauseous and the test is invalidated by vomiting. N.B. the current formulation of 73 Kcal carbohydrate/100 mL gives 75g glucose in 419 mL.

• Children: the dose is weight related – 1.75g/kg body weight: the maximum load is 75g.

Procedure
Blood samples (1-2 mL in fluoride oxalate tubes) should be taken in the fasting state and 120 min after consumption of the glucose load. There is no need to take urine samples for glucose measurements, nor blood at intermediate times.

Interpretation

	Plasma glucose (mmol/L)	
	0 min	120 min
Normal	< 6.1	< 7.8
Impaired glucose tolerance	6.1-6.9	7.8 - 11.0
Diabetic	≥ 7.0	≥ 11.1

Oral GTT for the diagnosis of growth hormone excess

Indication
Clinical suspicion of acromegaly or gigantism. Baseline GH values cannot be used to exclude acromegaly since elevated GH may occur with stress and low values (< 5 mU/L) are seen in up to 8% of acromegalic patients who are subsequently identified by the failure of GH to suppress during GTT.

Contraindications
This test is unnecessary in diabetic patients who should already have a suppressed GH in the presence of hyperglycaemia.

Principle
GH secretion is part of the counter-regulatory defence against hypoglycaemia; physiological GH secretion is inhibited by hyperglycaemia. In acromegaly and gigantism, GH secretion is autonomous and does not suppress. It may, paradoxically, rise with hyperglycaemia.

Side effects
Some subjects feel nauseated and may have vaso-vagal symptoms during this test.

Preparation
Patients should be advised to fast for 10-16 h prior to this test but may drink small volumes of water.

Requirements
- Adults: 75g anhydrous glucose in cold water. The solution should be chilled to improve palatability.

Lucozade ® is preferable to pure glucose solutions as it is less likely to make patients nauseous and the test is invalidated by vomiting. N.B. the current formulation of 73 Kcal carbohydrate/100 mL gives 75g glucose in 419 mL.

- Children: the dose is weight related - 1.75g/kg body weight: the maximum load is 75g.

- Indwelling cannula gauge 19.

- Five plain and five fluoride oxalate tubes.

Procedure

Insert an indwelling cannula and take blood samples for GH and glucose (1-2 mL in plain and 1-2 mL in fluoride oxalate tubes).

The glucose solution or Lucozade® should be drunk within five minutes. Take further blood samples for GH and glucose at 30, 60, 90 & 120 min.

Interpretation

Normal subjects will exhibit suppression of GH to undetectable values during the test.

NB: a paradoxical rise in GH may occur during GTT in normal adolescence.

Sensitivity and specificity

Fasting GH may be normal in 8% of acromegalic subjects but GH does NOT suppress to undetectable values during this test.

Reference

Brockmeier SJ, Buchfelder M, Adams EF, Schott W, Fahlbusch R. Acromegaly with 'normal' serum growth hormone levels. Horm Metab Res 1992; **24**: 392-6.

Gonadotrophin releasing hormone (GnRH) test

Indication
To diagnose hypothalamic-pituitary disease in precocious and delayed puberty in both sexes in children with low basal gonadotrophins concentrations.

Contraindications
This test may be performed simultaneously with the TRH and glucagon or insulin hypoglycaemia tests as part of a triple pituitary test.

Principle
GnRH (gonadotrophin releasing hormone) is a decapeptide secreted by the hypothalamus which stimulates the production and secretion of LH and FSH by the anterior pituitary.

Side effects
GnRH may rarely cause nausea, headache and abdominal pain.

Preparation
No specific patient preparation is required.

Requirements
- Three lithium heparin tubes.
- GnRH: the dose for children is 2.5 µg/kg body weight to a max 100µg.

Procedure

0 min	Take 3 mL blood for LH and FSH Immediately give GnRH i.v. as a bolus (dose as above)
20 min	Take 3 mL blood for LH and FSH
60 min	Take 3 mL blood for LH and FSH

Interpretation
Normal basal reference values in prepubertal children are:

       LH < 2.0 IU/L

       FSH < 2.0 IU/L

Following GnRH, the response may be considered normal if the basal values are in the reference range and there is at least a doubling at 20 min for both LH and FSH. The response varies throughout the menstrual cycle: early (day 4) < late follicular (day 11) = 'luteal' (day 21), max response occurs at the mid-cycle (day 14).

An exaggerated response is seen in primary and secondary gonadal failure.

A flat response in gonadotrophins (increase < 5 IU/L) occurs in prepubertal children and with pituitary and/or hypothalamic disease. However, a normal response does NOT exclude pituitary or hypothalamic disease since the response will be affected by the exact anatomy of the disorder.

The magnitude of the LH response is proportional to the mean nocturnal LH values and therefore the evolution of puberty.

References

Wu FCW, Butler GE, Kelnar CJH, Sellar RE. Patterns of pulsatile luteinizing hormone secretion before and during the onset of puberty in boys: a study using an immuno-radiometric assay. J Clin Endocrinol Metab 1990; **70:** 629-37.

Yen SSC, VandenBerg G, Rebar R, Ehara Y. Variations in pituitary response to synthetic LRF during different phases of the menstrual cycle. J Clin Endocrinol Metab 1972; **35:** 931-7.

hCG Stimulation Test

Indication
- In infants with ambiguous genitalia and palpable gonads.

- In males with delayed puberty and/or undescended testes.

- To confirm the presence of testes.

Male infants usually have plasma testosterone concentrations within the low adult range (8-12 nmol/L) during the third and fourth months. If blood can be obtained during this time, an hCG test may be avoided.

Contraindications
None.

Principle
hCG is a double polypeptide hormone and shares a common subunit with LH. It stimulates testicular Leydig cells to secrete androgens via the LH receptors. A single injection of hCG is adequate as it has a long half life (2.5 days) and produces a progressive but modest rise in plasma testosterone for 72-120 hours.

Side effects
Headaches, tiredness.

Preparation
No patient preparation is required.

Requirements
- One vial hCG 1500 units for infants or 5000 units for children over 2 years.

- Two plain blood tubes.

Procedure
Day 0: take blood for testosterone, androstenedione and dihydrotestosterone; administer 1500 units (infants) or 5000 units (over 2 yrs) hCG i.m.

Day 4: take blood for testosterone, androstenedione and dihydrotestosterone.

Interpretation

	Testosterone (nmol/L)	DHT (nmol/L)	T/DHT ratio before hCG	T/DHT ratio after hCG
Normal male adults	8-27	< 2.9	< 17	< 17
Normal male children (6 months - puberty)	< 0.9	< 0.1	< 20	< 27
5α-reductase deficiency (6 months - puberty)	< 0.5		< 20	> 27

There is a 2-9 fold increase in testosterone in normal prepubertal boys. In the absence of testes, no response in testosterone occurs.

References

Chaussain JC, Gendrel D, Roger M, Boudailleiz B, Job JC. Longitudinal study of plasma testosterone in male pseudohermaphroditism during early infancy. J Clin Endocrinol Metab 1979; **49:** 305-6.

Forest MG, Cathiard AM. Patterns of plasma testosterone and androstenedione in normal new-borns: evidence for testicular activity at birth. J Clin Endocrinol Metab 1975; **41:** 977-80.

Forest MG, David M, Lecoq A, Jeune M, Bertrans J. Kinetics of the hCG-induced steroidogenic response of the human testis. III. studies in children of the plasma levels of testosterone and hCG: rationale for testicular stimulation test. Pediatr Res 1980; **14:** 819-24.

Grant DB, Lawrence BM, Atherden SM, Ryness J. hCG stimulation test in children with abnormal sexual development. Arch Dis Child 1976; **51:** 596-601.

Saez JM, Forest MG. Kinetics of human chorionic gonadotropin-induced steroidogenic response of the human testis. 1. plasma testosterone: implications for human chorionic gonadotropin stimulation test. J Clin Endocrinol Metab 1979; **49:** 278-83.

Toscano V, Balducci R, Adama MV, Manca Bitti ML, Sciarra F, Boscherini B. Response to a single dose of human chorionic gonadotropin in prepubertal boys. Clin Endocrinol (Oxf) 1983; **57:** 421-4.

Hypertonic saline infusion

> This test is potentially dangerous and must be undertaken with great care
>
> Patients unable to conserve water may rapidly become critically hypertonic during this test

Indication
To make a clear diagnosis of cranial diabetes insipidus in subjects with polyuria and normal plasma osmolality.

Contraindications
Patients with epilepsy, cerebral or cardiovascular disease.

Principle
The test is designed to stress the integrity of the hypothalamo-renal (antidiuretic hormone (ADH)) axis. The infusion of hypertonic saline raises plasma osmolality and ensures maximal stimulation of ADH secretion. Failure of maximal renal concentration of urine itself does not differentiate between a defect in ADH secretion and one of renal response. The diagnosis can be seen by comparing the response of plasma ADH to plasma osmolality using the Newcastle chart.

Side effects
There is a serious risk of dehydration in patients with diabetes insipidus.

The hypertonic saline may induce thrombophlebitis at the site of infusion.

Preparation
Fast patient from midnight before the day of the test. Allow water only to be drunk until time of test (maximum volume 500 mL). No tea, coffee, alcohol or smoking after midnight. Patients should continue on any hormone replacement therapy.

Requirements
• Sphygmomanometer.
• Infusion pump and IV sets.
• 5% saline (500 - 1000 mL).
• Accurate scales for weighing the patient.
• Measuring cylinder (200 mL) for measuring urine volumes.
• Eight lithium heparin blood sample tubes and syringes cooled on ice.
• Eight urine sample bottles.

Procedure:

** Discuss with the laboratory on the day before the test **

1. Patient instructed to empty bladder. Measure urine volume and osmolality.
2. Weigh patient.
3. Patient to lie supine.
4. Insert cannula into antecubital veins of both arms, one for infusions, the other for blood sampling. Allow patient to rest for 30 min.
5. Take blood into chilled lithium heparin tube.
6. Repeat blood sample after 15 min.
7. Begin infusion of 5% saline at 0.04 mL/kg/min for 2 hours into non-blood-sampling arm.
8. Take blood samples at 30 min intervals.
9. Measure volume and osmolality of all urine passed.

Note time at which thirst is noted – if patient becomes very thirsty during test, give ice chips.

10. Take final blood sample 15 min after completion of infusion.
11. Record blood pressure, urine volume, blood sampling, patient's comments.
12. Allow patient to drink after test. Avoid ingestion of large fluid volumes.

Interpretation

Patients with primary polydipsia or nephrogenic diabetes insipidus have normal ADH release in response to the hyperosmolar state induced by this procedure. Patients with cranial diabetes insipidus have little or no rise in ADH.

Patients with nephrogenic diabetes insipidus have high plasma ADH with little or no concentration of urine i.e. urine osmolality < 300 mmol/kg.

References

Baylis PH. Robertson GL. Plasma vasopressin response to hypertonic saline infusion to assess posterior pituitary function. J Roy Soc Med (Lond) 1980; **73:** 255-60.

Baylis PH, Phillips EMG. The endocrine investigation of disorders of sodium and water homeostasis. J Int Fed Clin Chem 1994; **6:** 158-64.

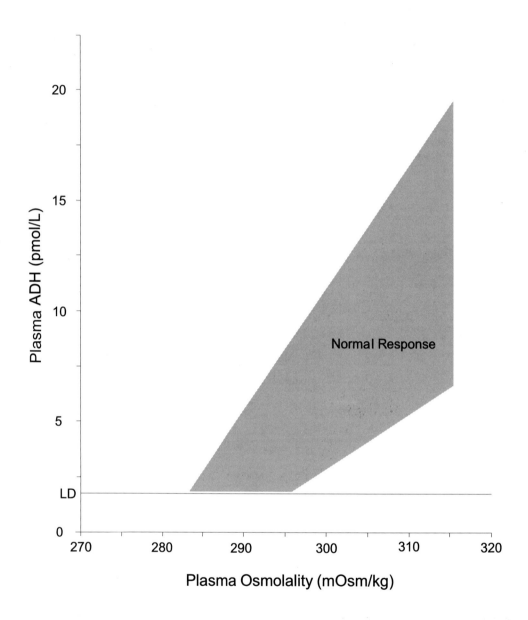

Newcastle chart (courtesy of Professor PH Bayliss)

Insulin hypoglycaemia test (IHT)

> This test is potentially dangerous and must be undertaken with great care.
> A DOCTOR OR NURSE MUST BE IN ATTENDANCE AT ALL TIMES.

Indication
Assessment of GH and ACTH/cortisol reserve. Differentiation of Cushing's syndrome from pseudo-Cushing's syndromes e.g. depression, alcohol excess.

Contraindications
- Age > 60 years.
- This test should not be performed on children outside a specialist paediatric endocrine unit.
- Ischaemic heart disease.
- Epilepsy.
- Severe panhypopituitarism, hypoadrenalism (09:00 cortisol < 100 nmol/L).
- Hypothyroidism impairs the GH and cortisol response. Patients should have corticosteroid replacement commenced prior to thyroxine as the latter has been reported to precipitate an Addisonian crisis in patients with dual deficiency. If adrenal insufficiency is confirmed, the need for a repeat IHT may need to be reconsidered after 3 months of thyroxine therapy.

Principle
ACTH and GH are both released as a part of the stress mechanism triggered by hypoglycaemia.

Side effects
Sweating, palpitation, loss of consciousness and, rarely, convulsions due to severe hypoglycaemia. Once hypoglycaemia has occurred, pituitary stimulation will have occurred and i.v. glucose should be given if severe symptoms are present. An Addisonian crisis may be precipitated in subjects with no adrenal reserve.

Preparation
The patient should fast overnight (water permitted) and be recumbent during the test.

An ECG must be normal and the patient should be weighed.

The side effects of the test should be clearly explained to the patient.

Requirements

- 50 mL 50% dextrose available for immediate administration for hypoglycaemia.
- Glucose test strips and lancets.
- Indwelling cannula gauge 19.
- Six fluoride and six plain tubes.

See protocol for emergency treatment of hypoglycaemia during IHT.
Actrapid insulin dose:

    0.15 U/kg for subjects with normal pituitary function
    0.10 U/kg for hypopituitary subjects
    0.2-0.3 U/kg for subjects with acromegaly, diabetes or Cushing's syndrome

Procedure

Site an indwelling cannula in the antecubital fossa with good access for administration of glucose, if required.

0 min	Take 3 mL blood in plain tubes for GH, cortisol and 1 mL in fluoride tube for glucose; inject insulin i.v.
30, 45, 60, 90, 120 min	Take 3 mL blood in plain tubes for GH, cortisol and 1 mL in fluoride tube for glucose

If there have been no clinical signs of hypoglycaemia by 45 min, the dose of insulin should be repeated and the test continued with blood samples timed again from 0 min.

Adequate hypoglycaemia (< 2.2 mmol/L) should be symptomatic. Record symptoms in the notes.

There must be at least two specimens following adequate hypoglycaemia.

Hypoglycaemia should be reversed if there are severe symptoms i.e. loss of consciousness, cardiac symptoms, extreme anxiety or fits. If necessary, i.v. 50% dextrose 0.4 mL/kg (i.e. 28 mL for a 70 kg adult) should be administered and blood sampling continued.

Once the test is completed, the subject should be given a supervised meal.

The subject should not drive for at least two hours after the test.

Interpretation

The test cannot be interpreted unless hypoglycaemia (blood glucose concentration < 2.2 mmol/L) is achieved.

Hypopituitarism: An adequate cortisol response is defined as a rise in plasma concetration to greater than 550 nmol/L. Patients with impaired cortisol responses i.e. maximum concentration < 550 but > 400 nmol/L may only need steroid cover for major illnesses or stresses. An increase in GH concentration to > 20 mU/L indicates normal pituitary GH reserve.

Cushing's syndrome: There is a rise of less than 170 nmol/L above the basal concentrations of cortisol.

Sensitivity and specificity

If there is adequate hypoglycaemia and the patient is not hypothyroid then the cortisol response is a good test of ACTH/adrenal reserve. However, 5-15% of normal subjects will show a suboptimal response as defined by maximum cortisol concentration < 550 nmol/L.

20% of patients with Cushing's syndrome will show a rise greater than 170 nmol/L. A rise of less than this is rare in depression or alcoholic pseudo-Cushing's syndromes which are the principal differential diagnoses.

References

Greenwood FC, Landon J, Stamp TCB. The plasma sugar, free fatty acid, cortisol and growth hormone response to insulin. 1. in control subjects. J Clin Invest 1965; **45:** 429-36.

Plumpton FS, Besser GM. The adrenocortical response to surgery and insulin-induced hypoglycaemia in corticosteroid-treated and normal subjects. Br J Surg 1969; **56:** 216-9.

Protocol for the emergency treatment of hypoglycaemia during the insulin hypoglycaemia or glucagon tests

Indication

This procedure is a guide to the treatment of children who become symptomatically hypoglycaemic, confirmed by a blood glucose < 2.5 mmol/L, during or after a glucagon test, or during an insulin tolerance test. The following equipment should be immediately available during the test procedure:

- liquid drink (squash/milk)
- food (toast/biscuits)
- glucose powder
- strong oral glucose solution (for diabetics)
- 10% dextrose (500 mL) and i.v. giving set
- glucose meter, strips and lancets
- hydrocortisone 100 mg for i.v. use.

Emergency treatment

IF THE CHILD REMAINS CONSCIOUS

Give a drink of milk/squash with 2-4 teaspoons of dextrose dissolved in it. If this is not successful, give 5-20 mL strong dextrose solution ORALLY. In most instances this will be sufficient to raise the blood glucose over 2 mmol/L. DO NOT ABANDON THE TEST AT THIS STAGE

IF THE CHILD BECOMES UNCONSCIOUS

Do not attempt oral therapy. Abandon the test procedure.
Give intravenous glucose 200 mg/kg (10% dextrose at 2 mL/kg) over 3 minutes.

Emergency i.v. 10% glucose bolus dose

Weight	Total volume
10 kg	20 mL
15 kg	30 mL
20 kg	40 mL
30 kg	60 mL

and continue with 10% glucose infusion i.v. at a rate of 10 mg/kg/min (0.1 mL/kg/min) until the child becomes sufficiently conscious to take oral fluids

i.v. 10% glucose infusion dose after bolus

Weight	Infusion rate
10 kg	1 mL/min or 60 mL/h
15 kg	1.5 mL/min or 90 mL/h
20 kg	2 mL/min or 120 mL/h
30 kg	3 mL/min or 180 mL/h

Ischaemic exercise test

Indication

This test is useful in the differential diagnosis of metabolic causes of muscle weakness, fatigue and cramps e.g. disorders of glycolysis and myoadenylate deaminase deficiency. These disorders should be considered in all patients who complain of muscle cramps and exercise intolerance.

Contraindications

There are anecdotal reports of the development of rhabdomyolysis if patients with underlying acquired (e.g. alcoholic or hypothyroid) or inherited myopathies are strenuously exercised.

Principle of the test

Normal subjects will exhibit a rise in both plasma lactate and ammonia concentrations during ischaemic exercise. Further metabolism of lactate does not occur during ischaemic exercise since oxygen is required for further metabolism in the tricarboxylic acid (TCA) cycle. Ammonia rises as a result of amino acid deamination by myoadenylate deaminase to provide substrates for the TCA cycle. Intact pathways are required for such rises in lactate and ammonia.

Side effects

This test is uncomfortable/painful to perform and subjects will need encouragement to ensure that sufficient exercise is performed for a valid test.

Preparation

The subject should rest for 30 min prior to the test.

Requirements

- Six lithium heparin tubes for ammonia.
- Six special tubes for lactate (discuss with laboratory).
- Ice for sample transport.
- Sphygmomanometer.
- Saline or Hepsal® for maintaining cannulae patency.

Procedure

At each time point samples should be taken for lactate (1 mL) and ammonia (1 mL). The tubes for ammonia should be kept on ice and transported to the laboratory as soon as possible

A sphygmomanometer cuff is placed on the upper arm and an intravenous cannula inserted in the antecubital vein which should be kept patent with Hepsal®. A baseline blood sample is drawn from the occluded arm. The cuff is inflated above systolic pressure and the subject squeezes the sphygmomanometer bulb once every second for 1 minute or until the onset of muscle fatigue. Affected subjects are usually unable to perform this work for more than 40-50 seconds. After one minute ischaemia the cuff is deflated. Further blood samples are taken from the occluded arm 1, 2, 3, 5 and 7 min after deflating the cuff.

Interpretation
Normal subjects obtain relatively instantaneous relief of pain and can move their fingers immediately on release of the cuff. Patients with metabolic defects often cannot exercise for two minutes, develop marked forearm contracture, and are unable to extend their fingers.

A normal response is shown by maximum rises in both plasma lactate (to > 2.2 mmol/L) and in plasma ammonia (to > 70 µmol/L) concentrations. A normal increment in one analyte alone does not exclude disease. A failure of both lactate and ammonia to rise suggests that the subject did not exercise adequately and the test should be repeated. The absence of a venous lactate response to ischaemic exercise is characteristic of all diseases in which there is an impairment in the conversion of glycogen to glucose or glucose to lactate in muscle. The absence of a rise in ammonia with a normal lactate rise is characteristic of myoadenylate deaminase deficiency.

Sensitivity and specificity
Failure of lactate to rise after this test confirms a diagnosis of a disorder of glycolysis but this test cannot be used to exclude partial expression of these diseases.

References
Coleman RA, Stajich JM, Pact VW, Pericak-Vance MA. The ischemic exercise test in normal adults and in patients with weakness and cramps. Muscle & nerve 1986; **9:** 216-21.

Kanbe K, Nagase M, Udagawa E. Acute alcoholic rhabdomyolysis associated with abnormal ischemic exercise test. Muscle & nerve 1993; **16:** 1269-70.

Riggs JE. Acute exertional rhabdomyolysis in hypothyroidism: the result of a reversible defect in glycogenolysis. Militar Med 1990; **155:** 171-2.

Taylor RG, Lieberman JS, Portwood MM. Ischemic exercise test: failure to detect partial expression of McArdle's disease. Muscle & nerve 1987; **10:** 546-51.

Magnesium infusion for the investigation and treatment of magnesium deficiency

Indication
Magnesium deficiency is often considered the 'forgotten anion' in view of the magnitude of unrecognised deficiency in hospital inpatients (approximately 10%). This test is only rarely required, for example when signs of magnesium deficiency occur with borderline low plasma magnesium concentrations. Oral replacement therapy for the majority of patients does not need to be assessed.

Contraindication
This loading dose of magnesium should not be given in subjects with renal failure, cardiac dysrhythmias or respiratory failure. It should not be performed unless causes of renal loss have been excluded (alcoholism, salt-losing nephropathy, hyperaldosteronism, glycosuria, etc.) nor in subjects who are taking drugs which affect tubular function (diuretics, cisplatin, cyclosporin, etc.).

Principle
Magnesium is predominantly an intracellular ion with less than 1% being in the extracellular compartment. Plasma or erythrocyte magnesium concentrations are therefore relatively poor indicators of body magnesium status. This loading test measures the retention of magnesium and therefore reflects the degree of deficiency.

Side effects
Tiredness, sensation of heat and occasionally mild generalised redness of the skin.

Preparation
No specific patient preparation is required.

Requirements
- 30 mmol magnesium in 500 mL 5% dextrose for intravenous administration.
- 24 h urine bottle.

Procedure
Administer the magnesium intravenously over 12 h. Collect all urine passed over the 24 h period following the onset of magnesium infusion.

Interpretation
Magnesium depletion is unlikely if more than 24 mmol magnesium are excreted in the 24 h collection. Normal subjects retain less than 10% of infused load.

Patients with acute myocardial infarction, with chronic ischaemic heart disease or on diuretics have been demonstrated to have mild magnesium deficiency as they retain more magnesium. Such patients will excrete less than 20 mmol in the 24 h urine collection.

References

Dyckner T, Wester PO. Magnesium deficiency - guidelines for diagnosis and substitution therapy. Acta Med Scand 1982; **suppl 661:** 37-41.

Gullestad L, Midtvedt K, Dolva LO, Norseth J, Kjekshus J. The magnesium loading test: reference values in healthy subjects. Scand J Clin Lab Invest 1994; **54:** 23-31.

Rasmussen HS, McNair P, Goransson L, Belslor S, Larsen OG, Aurup P. Magnesium deficiency in patients with ischaemic heart disease with and without acute myocardial infarction uncovered by an intravenous magnesium loading test. Arch Int Med 1988; **148:** 329-32.

Pituitary function tests for children

Indication

Pituitary function tests are often requested in the diagnostic evaluation of short children. The aim under these circumstances is to determine the status of the growth hormone (GH) axis. However, a prolonged test of GH secretion with multiple blood samples is an invasive procedure and in order to reduce the need for repeat investigation, it has been traditional to include the use of TRH and GnRH. Recent data suggests that additional stimulation with TRH and GnRH does not provide any information that would not have been given by baseline measurements of gonadotrophins, sex hormones, TSH and thyroxine.

Our practice is to use the glucagon test (see page .142..) for evaluation of growth hormone and cortisol secretion and to include TRH and GnRH only if there is a specific indication for these tests.

Contraindications

See individual tests.

Principle

See individual tests.

Side effects

There is a greater risk of hypoglycaemia in children as they have smaller reserves of fat and carbohydrate and therefore, contingency plans must be available for its development. Most subjects given glucagon experience nausea and some may vomit.

Preparation

This test must be performed at least 4 h after any food and drink.

Requirements

The following equipment should be immediately available: see protocol for emergency treatment of hypoglycaemia during IHT/glucagon test (page 160).

- Liquid drink (squash/milk), food (toast/biscuits).
- Glucose powder, strong oral glucose solution (as for diabetics).
- 10% dextrose (500 mL) and i.v. giving set.
- Glucose test strips and lancets.
- Hydrocortisone 100 mg for i.v. use.
- Seven plain and seven fluoride tubes.
- An intravenous cannula.

Drugs given as separate boluses TRH and GnRH only if specifically indicated - see Indication	Glucagon 15 µg/kg by i.m.injection, maximum 1 mg TRH 7 µg/kg i.v., maximum 200 µg GnRH 2.5 µg/kg i.v., maximum 100 µg

Procedure

0 min	Take 3 mL blood for TSH, LH, FSH, cortisol and GH and 1 mL in fluoride tube for glucose. Immediately give glucagon, TRH and GnRH
30, 60, 90, 120, 150 and 180 min	Take 3 mL blood for cortisol and GH

Interpretation
See glucagon test for hypothalamo-pituitary axis (page 142).

The use of seven samples is required for children whereas only three are required for aduts as the peaks for cortisol and growth hormone occur earlier.

Reference
Burke CW. The pituitary megatest: outdated? Clin Endocrinol (Oxf) 1992; **36:** 133-4.

Westwood ME, Butler GE, Mclellan AC, Barth JH. The combined pituitary function test in children: an evaluation of the clinical usefulness of TRH and LHRH stimulation tests through a retrospective analysis of one hundred and twenty six cases. Clin Endocrinol (Oxf) 2000; **52:** 727-33.

Penicillamine test for the diagnosis of Wilson's disease

Indication
The diagnosis of Wilson's disease is difficult and should be made on a combination of investigations including serum copper (< 12 μmol/L) and caeruloplasmin concentration (< 0.2 g/L), and 24 h urine copper excretion (> 1.2 μmol). Some authorities believe that the copper concentration of liver tissue is the most important criterion but this may be compromised by the inherent difficulty in obtaining both appropriate reference material and adequate patient samples. Despite these investigations, the diagnosis of Wilson's disease may not be clearcut and the test described may be of further use.

Contraindication
Known allergy to penicillamine.

The use of penicillamine prior to the investigation will compromise this test since it will have reduced the copper stores. Since the extent to which the stores will have been depleted is unknown, it would be prudent to avoid using this test within six months of penicillamine use.

Principle
Penicillamine solubilises copper and allows the stores to be excreted in the urine.

Side effects
Some patients may have an allergic reaction to penicillamine.

Preparation
No special preparation required.

Requirements
- Plain tube for blood sample.
- Three 24 h urine containers with no preservatives.
- Two 500 mg penicillamine tabs.

Procedure
At least two baseline measurements of 24 h urinary copper should be made prior to this test.

09:00 h	Take 10 mL blood in plain tube for serum copper and caeruloplasmin Start 24 h urine collection for copper Administer 500 mg d-penicillamine
21:00 h	Administer a second dose of 500 mg d-penicillamine
09:00 h	Complete 24 h urine collection

Interpretation

The diagnosis of Wilson's disease should always be considered since the diagnostic accuracy of measurements of copper metabolism may be compromised by the presence of liver failure. The following threshold values are guidelines for Wilson's disease and a combination of abnormal results is probably necessary for a diagnosis to be made.

Caeruloplasmin	< 0.2 g/L
Serum copper	< 12 µmol/L
Urine copper	> 4 µmol/24h
Urine copper post-penicillamine	> 25 µmol/24h

Sensitivity and specificity

Low serum caeruloplasmin may be seen in malnutrition, malabsorption and nephrotic syndrome as well as all forms of chronic liver disease especially primary biliary cirrhosis; low serum copper may be disguised by an increase of up to 30% in inflammatory states.

If equivocal results are obtained from the penicillamine test, the next investigative step is to biopsy the liver to measure tissue copper content. This is so useful that some authorities believe that a liver copper measurement should be made on all diagnostic liver biopsies.

Reference

da Costa DM, Baldwin D, Portmann B, Lolin Y, Mowat A, Mieli-Vergani G. Value of urinary copper excretion after penicillamine challenge in the diagnosis of Wilson's disease. Hepatology 1992; **15:** 609-15.

Short Synacthen test for suspected adrenal failure

Indication
This is performed for the investigation of adrenal insufficiency. There is no evidence to support the use of this test in the management of steroid replacement or withdrawal.

Contraindication
The Synacthen test gives unreliable results in the two weeks following pituitary surgery. It should be noted that prednisilone crossreacts with cortisol assays.

Principle
Adrenal glucocorticoid secretion is controlled by adrenocorticotrophic hormone (ACTH) released by the anterior pituitary. This test evaluates the ability of the adrenal cortex to produce cortisol after stimulation by synthetic ACTH (tetracosactrin: Synacthen). It does not test the pituitary-adrenal axis.

Side effects
There are rare reports of hypersensitivity reactions to Synacthen, particularly in children with a history of allergic disorders.

Preparation
There are no dietary restrictions for this test. This test should be performed in the morning as the cortisol responses between the morning and late afternoon may differ by as much as 100 nmol/L 30 min post Synacthen.

Requirements
- Two plain tubes.
- 250 µg Synacthen (1 vial).
- The dose for children is 36 µg/kg body weight up to a maximum of 250 µg.

Procedure

09:00 h	Take 3 mL blood for cortisol Inject Synacthen i.v. or i.m.
09:30 h	Take 3 mL blood for cortisol

Interpretation
1. Adrenal insufficiency is excluded by a rise in cortisol of > 200 nmol/L and a 30 min

value > 600 nmol/L.

2. The above definition only defines adrenal insufficiency. The definition of normality is problematic since there is considerable variation in healthy individuals and a significant overlap with patients who have adrenal insufficiency.

3. In ACTH deficiency the response to the short test may be normal or reduced.

4. The response to Synacthen is not affected by obesity.

5. There is no difference in cortisol response between i.v. and i.m. administration.

6. Baseline and post-Synacthen cortisol values do NOT apply to women taking oral contraceptives.

Sensitivity and specificity
There are reports of patients with incipient adrenal failure with normal responses to Synacthen. The use of physiological doses e.g. 5 µg may prove more useful at determining those subjects with poor responses than conventional (250 µg) pharmacological doses.

References
Azziz R, Zacur HA, Parker CR Jr, Bradley EL Jr, Boots LR. Effect of obesity on the response to acute adrenocorticotropin stimulation in eumenorrhoeic women. Fertil Steril 1991; **56:** 427-33.

Clarke PMS, Neylon I, Raggatt PR, Sheppard MC, Stewart PM. Defining the normal cortisol response to the short Synacthen test: implications for the investigation of hypothalamo-pituitary disorders. Clin Endocrinol (Oxf) 1998; **49:** 287-92.

Ostlere LS, Rumsby G, Holownia P, Jacobs HS, Rustin HA, Honour JW. Carrier status for steroid 21-hydroxylase deficiency is only one factor in the variable phenotype of acne. Clin Endocrinol (Oxf) 1998; **48:** 209-15.

Patel SR, Selby C, Jeffcoate WJ. The short synacthen test in acute hospital admissions. Clin Endocrinol (Oxf) 1991; **35:** 259-61.

Reingold A, Guillemant S, Ghata NJ, Guillemant J, Touitou Y, Dupont W, Lagoguey M, Bourgeois P, Briere L, Fraboulet G, Guillet P. Clinical chronopharmacology of ACTH 1-17. 1 effects on plasma cortisol and urinary 17-hydroxycorticosteroids. Chronobiologica 1980; **17:** 513-23.

Depot (prolonged) Synacthen test

Indication
This is performed for the differentiation of primary from secondary adrenal failure. The ready availability of ACTH assays may now make this test protocol redundant.

Contraindications
The Synacthen test gives unreliable results in the two weeks following pituitary surgery.

Principle
The long Synacthen test was designed to confirm the diagnosis of primary adrenal failure. The diagnosis of adrenal failure is made on the basis of the cortisol response to ACTH at 30 min (see short Synacthen test). The prolonged stimulation of the adrenals by ACTH in the long Synacthen test results in a degree of recovery by adrenal glands which may have become atrophic due to pituitary failure, whereas when the adrenal glands are themselves diseased they cannot respond.

Side effects
There are rare reports of hypersensitivity reactions to 'Synacthen' particularly in children with a history of allergic disorders.

Preparation
There are no dietary restrictions for this test. However, those patients who are already taking corticosteroids should have been taking them for less than two weeks and should be switched to dexamethasone 24 hours before the test.

Requirements
- Six plain tubes.
- 1 mg Depot Synacthen (1 vial).

Procedure

09:00 h	Take 3 mL blood for cortisol Inject Synacthen 250 µg i.v. Take further blood samples for cortisol at 1, 2, 4, 8 and 24 hours

Interpretation

Time	95% confidence interval cortisol responses in normal subjects
1 h	605 - 1265 nmol/L
2 h	750 - 1520 nmol/L
4 h	960 - 1650 nmol/L
8 h	1025 - 1600 nmol/L
24 h	610 - 1500 nmol/L

A gradual rise with a peak cortisol response at 4 - 8 hours occurs in normal subjects. A failure to respond, or an initial response at 60 min which is not sustained, indicates primary adrenal failure.

A response that rises gradually to a peak at 24 hours occurs in secondary adrenal failure i.e. due to pituitary failure or prolonged corticosteroid therapy. Some cases of long-standing adrenal atrophy will not respond even after 24 hours and may require several daily doses of depot Synacthen before an adrenal response is seen. The majority of these latter cases should be identifiable by measurement of plasma ACTH.

References
Galvao-Teles A, Burke CW, Fraser TR. Adrenal function tested with tetracosactrin depot. Lancet 1971; **i:** 557-60.

Jenkins RC, Ross RJM. Protocols for common endocrine tests. In: Grossman A (ed). Clinical Endocrinology. Blackwells Science, Oxford. 2nd edit 1998: 1117-34.

Short Synacthen test for CAH

Indication
This is performed for the diagnosis of congenital adrenal hyperplasia (CAH) due to 21-hydroxylase deficiency in children and adults. This test is often carried out in hyperandrogenised women to diagnose late-onset CAH. However, the diagnosis of this condition does not affect treatment nor does it appear to indicate a risk of cortisol deficiency during physioogical crises.

Contraindication
The Synacthen test gives unreliable results in the two weeks following pituitary surgery.

Principle
Adrenal glucocorticoid secretion is controlled by adrenocorticotrophic hormone (ACTH) released by the anterior pituitary. This test evaluates the ability of the adrenal cortex to produce cortisol after stimulation by synthetic ACTH (tetracosactrin: Synacthen). In subjects with enzyme deficiency in the steroid synthetic pathway, cortisol may, or may not, be adequately secreted. However, there is excessive secretion of the precursor steroids before the defective enzyme. The commonest form of CAH is due to deficiency of 21-hydroxylase and in these subjects increased secretion of 17 OH-progesterone occurs.

Side effects
There are rare reports of hypersensitivity reactions to Synacthen particularly in children with a history of allergic disorders.

Preparation
There are no dietary restrictions for this test. This test should be performed in the morning as the cortisol responses between the morning and late afternoon may differ by as much as 100 nmol/L 30 min post-Synacthen.

Requirements
- Two plain tubes.
- 250 mg Synacthen (1 vial).
- The dose for children is 36 μg/kg body weight up to a maximum of 250 μg.

Procedure

09:00 h	Take 5 mL blood for cortisol and 17 OH-progesterone Inject Synacthen i.v.
09:30 h	Take 5 mL blood for cortisol and 17 OH-progesterone

Interpretation

A normal cortisol response is indicated by a rise in the cortisol concentration of the 30 min sample to greater than 600 nmol/L.

CAH is suggested by a baseline 17 OH-progesterone >12 nmol/L. A baseline of > 100 nmol/L is diagnostic of homozygosity for 21 OH-deficiency and the stimulation test is not required.

Heterozygotes for 21 OH-deficiency have post-ACTH values of 17 OH-progesterone > 35 nmol/L.

Adults with the rarer forms of late-onset CAH e.g. 3β-hydroxylase or 11-hydroxylase have normal 17 OH-progesterone responses to ACTH.

References

Eldar-Geva T, Hurwitz A, Vecsei P, Palti Z, Milwidsky A, Rosler A. Secondary biosynthetic defects in women with late-onset congenital adrenal hyperplasia. New Engl J Med 1990; **323:** 855-63.

New MI, Lorenzen F, Lerner AJ, Kohn B, Oberfield SE, Pollack MS, Dupont B, Stoner E, Levy DJ, Pang S, Levine LS. Genotyping steroid 21-hydroxylase deficiency: hormonal reference data. J Clin Endocrinol Metab 1983; **57:** 320-6

Thyrotropin releasing hormone (TRH) test

Indication
The development of TSH assays capable of accurate measurements below 0.1 mU/L has obviated the need for the TRH test in most cases of thyroid disease in adults except perhaps in the differential diagnosis of TSHoma and thyroid hormone resistance (high TSH and high thyroxine in both cases).

Contraindications
TRH can cause smooth muscle spasm and should be used with caution in patients with asthma or ischaemic heart disease. The TRH test should not be used in pregnant women. Patients should not have taken thyroxine or triiodothyronine for 3 weeks prior to this test.

Principle
TRH (thyrotropin releasing hormone) is a tripeptide secreted by the hypothalamus that stimulates the production and secretion of TSH by the anterior pituitary. TRH also stimulates prolactin release.

Side effects
Most adult patients express an urgent need but inability to pass urine. Other side effects include flushing, dizziness and a metallic taste in the mouth.

Preparation
No specific patient preparation is required.

Requirements
- Three plain tubes.
- TRH 200 µg (adults). The dose for children is 7 µg/kg body weight up to 200 µg.

Procedure

0 min	Take 3 mL blood for TSH Immediately give TRH i.v. as a bolus
20 min	Take 3 mL blood for TSH
60 min	Take 3 mL blood for TSH

Interpretation

Normal basal values of TSH should be 0.2-6.0 mU/L. The normal increment in TSH at 20 min should be 5-30 (mean 15) mU/L with a slight fall in concentration from the peak value at 60 min. Exaggerated TSH response is seen in primary hypothyroidism. A peak response less than 5 mU/L is seen in primary hyperthyroidism, but also in some apparently euthyroid patients with ophthalmic Graves' disease or multi-nodular goitre. A delayed response with the TSH concentration lower at 20 than 60 min may be seen in hypothalamic dysfunction, but is not a reliable indicator of this.

Various drugs can modify the TSH response. This is reduced by glucocorticoids, dopamine agonists e.g. l-DOPA, bromocriptine and fluoxetine; and enhanced by dopamine antagonists e.g. metoclopramide, oestrogens and theophylline and sertra-line.

In neonates, peak TSH responses < 35 mU/L are not associated with subsequent hypothyroidism, whereas responses > 35 mU/L are associated with a rate of subsequent hypothyroidism of 35%.

The TSH response is flat in most cases of TSHoma whereas in thyroid hormone resistance the TSH response is brisk.

References

Baylis PH. Drug induced endocrine disorders. Adverse Drug Reaction Bull 1986; **116:** 432-5.

Brucker-Davis F, Ildfield EH, Skarulis MC, Doppman JL, Weintraub BD. Thyrotropin-secreting pituitary tumours: diagnostic criteria, thyroid hormone sensitivity, and treatment outcome in 25 patients followed at the National Institutes of Health. J Clin Endocrinol Metab 1999; **84:** 476-486.

Casanueva FF, Webb SM, Dieguez C. Thyrotrophin-secreting pituitary tumours. In: Grossman A (ed). Clinical Endocrinology. Blackwell Science, 2nd edit 1997: 204-15.

Pijl H, Koppeschaar HP, Willekens FL, Frolich M, Meinders AE. The influence of serotonergic neurotransmission on pituitary hormone release in obese and non-obese females. Acta Endocrinologica 1993; **128:** 319-24.

Rapaport R, Sills I, Patel U, Oppenheimer E, Skuza K, Horlick M, Goldstein S, Dimartino J, Saenger P. Thyrotropin-releasing hormone stimulation in infants. J Clin Endocrinol Metab 1993; **77:** 889-94.

Water deprivation test 1: strongly suspected case of DI

This test is potentially dangerous and must be undertaken with great care. Patients unable to conserve water may become critically dehydrated within a few hours of water restriction.

Indication
Investigation of suspected cranial or nephrogenic diabetes insipidus and primary polydipsia

Contraindications
Other causes of polydipsia and polyuria e.g. diabetes mellitus, hypoadrenalism, hypercalcaemia, hypokalaemia, chronic renal failure and therapy with carbamazepine, chlorpropamide or lithium.

The test is not required if there is evidence for the ability to concentrate urine e.g. spot urine osmolality > 750 mmoL/kg.

Principle of test
Water restriction in the normal individual results in secretion of ADH by the posterior pituitary in order to reclaim water from the distal renal tubules. Failure of this mechanism results in a rise in plasma osmolality owing to water loss, and a dilute urine of low osmolality. The two causes are a failure of ADH secretion and insensitivity of the renal tubules to ADH. They may be distinguished by the administration of DDAVP (synthetic ADH).

Side effects
Patients with true diabetes insipidus may become severely water depleted during water deprivation and MUST be carefully monitored throughout the procedure.

Preparation
DO NOT RESTRICT FLUIDS UNTIL THE TEST COMMENCES

Requirements
• Accurate weighing scales for weighing the patient.
• Measuring cylinders for measuring hourly urine volumes.

Procedure

08:00 h	Weigh subject and begin fluid balance chart. Calculate and record 95% of initial body weight. Take samples of urine and blood for osmolality.
09:00 h -	Commence fluid restriction Hourly weigh the subject, measure urine volume and osmolality

FLUID RESTRICTION SHOULD BE STOPPED IF:

• There is a fall in weight of > 5% *or*

• Plasma osmolality increases to > 300mOsm/kg

These values indicate a degree of dehydration which should never be reached with careful observation of the subject.

Proceed to DDAVP test if urine osmolality rises by < 30 mmol/kg (*in toto*) over 3 successive urine samples. The test should be terminated if urine osmolality rises to > 750 mmol/kg.

Post-dehydration osmolality (mmol/kg)		Post-DDAVP osmolality (mmol/kg)	Diagnosis
Plasma	Urine	Urine	
283 - 293	> 750	> 750	Normal
> 293	< 300	< 300	Nephrogenic diabetes insipidus
> 293	< 300	> 750	Cranial diabetes insipidus
< 293	300-750	< 750	Chronic polydipsia
< 293	300-750	> 750	Partial nephrogenic DI or primary polydipsia

Interpretation

NB: chronic primary polydipsia can dilute the renal medullary osmotic gradient, thereby reducing the renal response to endogenous and exogenous ADH. In cranial DI, maximal urinary concentration may be achieved only after repeated DDAVP.

Sensitivity and specificity

The water deprivation test has a sensitivity and specificity of 95% for diagnosing and differentiating severe cranial DI and nephrogenic DI. The incidence of false positive and false negative results for primary polydipsia or partial CDI/NDI is 30-40% and then patients may need further investigation (see flow chart for polyuria - page 52).

References

Thompson CJ. Polyuric states in man. Clin Endocrinol Metab 1989; **3:** 473-97.

Miller M, Dalakos T, Moses AM, Fellerman H, Streeten DHP. Recognition of partial defects in antidiuretic hormone secretion. Arch Intern Med 1970; **73:** 721-9.

Water deprivation test 2: DI not strongly suspected

This test is potentially dangerous and must be undertaken with great care. Patients unable to conserve water may become critically dehydrated within a few hours of water restriction

Indication
If DI is not strongly suspected or if the level 1 test was uninterpretable i.e. not continued for long enough, or if there is already evidence that the kidneys have some concentrating ability e.g. random urine osmolality > plasma, then it is safe to proceed to the modified water deprivation test.

Contraindications
Other causes of polydipsia and polyuria e.g. diabetes mellitus, hypoadrenalism, hypercalcaemia, hypokalaemia, chronic renal failure and therapy with carbamazepine, chlorpropamide or lithium therapy.

The test is not required if there is evidence for the ability to concentrate urine e.g. spot urine osmolality > 750 mmol/kg.

Principle of test
Water restriction in the normal individual results in secretion of ADH by the posterior pituitary in order to reclaim water from the distal renal tubules. Failure of this mechanism results in a rise in plasma osmolality owing to water loss, and a dilute urine of low osmolality. The two causes are a failure of ADH secretion and insensitivity of the renal tubules to ADH and they may be distinguished by the administration of DDAVP (synthetic ADH).

Side effects
Patients with true diabetes insipidus may become severely water depleted during water deprivation and MUST be carefully monitored throughout the procedure.

Preparation
Restrict food and drink after midnight prior to test.
Subjects should not smoke during the day of the test and should avoid alcohol and caffeine containing drinks on the previous evening (as alcohol caffeine and nicotine influence the action of ADH).

Requirements
- Accurate weighing scales for weighing the patient.
- Measuring cylinders for measuring hourly urine volumes.

00:00 h	Fluid restriction should commence
08:00 h	Weigh subject, measure urine volume and urine and plasma osmolality
09:00 h	Continue hourly with above urine measurements

Procedure

FLUID RESTRICTION SHOULD BE STOPPED IF:

- There is a fall in weight of > 5% *or*

- Plasma osmolality increases to > 300 mmol/kg.

These values indicate a degree of dehydration which should never be reached with careful observation of the subject.

Proceed to DDAVP test if urine osmolality rises < 30 mmol/kg (in toto) over 3 successive urine samples. The test should be terminated if urine osmolality rises > 750 mmol/kg.

Water deprivation test 3: DDAVP Test

Procedure
Administer DDAVP 2 mg i.m.

Measure urine volume and osmolality at hourly intervals for at least 3 hours.

Interpretation
See Water deprivation test 1

Sensitivity and Specificity
See Water deprivation test 1

References
Thompson CJ. Polyuric states in man. Clin Endocrinol Metab 1989; **3:** 473-497.

Miller M, Dalakos T, Moses AM, Fellerman H, Streeten DHP. Recognition of partial defects in antidiuretic hormone secretion. Arch Intern Med 1970; **73:** 721-729.